BECOMING AN ALZHEIMERS WHISPERER™

A RESOURCE FOR FAMILY CAREGIVERS

By: Verna Benner Carson, PhD, PMH/CNS-BC and Katherine J. Vanderhorst, R.N., B.S.N.

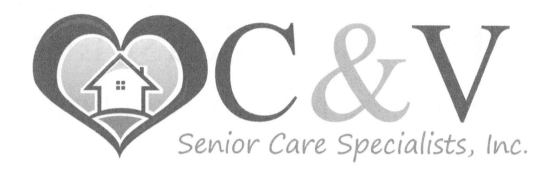

www.cvseniorcare.com

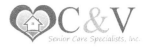

TABLE OF CONTENTS
Becoming an Alzheimer's Whisperer
A Resource for Family Caregivers

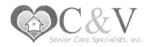

SECTION 5: SAFETY CONCERNS

Section 6: Challenging Behaviors

Section 7: Special Considerations

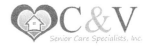

Dear Caregiver,

If you are reading this resource guide, than you are probably struggling to provide care to someone with Alzheimer's disease. Perhaps it is a loved one – husband, wife, mother, father, a grandparent, an in-law or another family member or you are a paid caregiver to someone with this disease. Whatever your relationship is to the person with the disease you are most likely encountering "care giving battles". Perhaps the person resists bathing and dressing not only with words but also with actions such as hitting, biting, kicking, spitting and pulling hair. You have reasoned, cajoled, argued with, yelled at, or even threatened this person – all without success. You are frustrated and overwhelmed! You are the person for whom we wrote this resource guide! Believe us when we say caregiving does not have to be a battle but can actually be fun and personally fulfilling.

Let us show you how!

Our Best...
Verna and Katherine

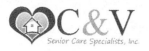

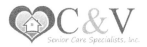

SECTION 1

LET'S GET STARTED WITH A FOCUS ON YOU THE CAREGIVER

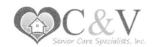

When you are involved in caregiving over a long period of time you gradually adjust to the demands made on you. You don't notice that you have given up friendships and activities that once gave you pleasure. You even postpone your own medical appointments because you "just don't have time". These changes don't happen all at once so you don't even realize how stressed and burdened you are. Responding to these easy questions might be an "eye-opener" for you that permits you to say, "I am overwhelmed and it is perfectly okay to accept help!"

CAREGIVER BURDEN SCALE

Caregivers often suffer burn-out because of the changes they must face in their everyday lives and routines. Caring for another-although rewarding, can be very difficult and demanding on a person's physical, emotional and spiritual well-being. The following statements reflect how people sometimes think when they are taking care of another person. After each question, indicate how often you think that way.

Never =0; Rarely =1; Sometimes =2; Frequently =3, or Nearly Always=4.

There are no right or wrong answers. Total your score to assess your level of burden.

1. **Do you think that your relative asks for more help than he or she needs?**
Never =0; Rarely =1; Sometimes =2; Frequently =3, or Nearly Always=4.
2. **Do you think that because of the time you spend with your relative, you do not have enough time for yourself?**
Never =0; Rarely =1; Sometimes =2; Frequently =3, or Nearly Always=4.
3. **Do you feel stressed between caring for your relative and trying to meet other responsibilities you do not have enough time for yourself?**
Never =0; Rarely =1; Sometimes =2; Frequently =3, or Nearly Always=4.
4. **Do you feel embarrassed over your relative's behavior?**
Never =0; Rarely =1; Sometimes =2; Frequently =3, or Nearly Always=4.
5. **Do you feel angry when you are around your relative?**
Never =0; Rarely =1; Sometimes =2; Frequently =3, or Nearly Always=4.
6. **Do you think that your relative currently affects your relationship with other family members or friends in a negative way?**
Never =0; Rarely =1; Sometimes =2; Frequently =3, or Nearly Always=4.
7. **Are you afraid about what the future holds for your relative?**
Never =0; Rarely =1; Sometimes =2; Frequently =3, or Nearly Always=4.
8. **Do you think your relative is dependent on you?**
Never =0; Rarely =1; Sometimes =2; Frequently =3, or Nearly Always=4.

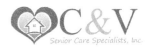

9. **Do you feel strained when you are around your relative?**
Never =0; Rarely =1; Sometimes =2; Frequently =3, or Nearly Always=4.

10. **Do you think your health has suffered because of your involvement with your relative?**
Never =0; Rarely =1; Sometimes =2; Frequently =3, or Nearly Always=4.

11. **Do you feel that you do not have as much privacy as you would like, because of your relative?**
Never =0; Rarely =1; Sometimes =2; Frequently =3, or Nearly Always=4.

12. **Do you think your social life has suffered because you are caring for your relative?**
Never =0; Rarely =1; Sometimes =2; Frequently =3, or Nearly Always=4.

13. **Do you feel uncomfortable having friends over because of your relative?**
Never =0; Rarely =1; Sometimes =2; Frequently =3, or Nearly Always=4.

14. **Do you think that your relative expects you to take care of him/her as if you were the only one he/she can depend on?**
Never =0; Rarely =1; Sometimes =2; Frequently =3, or Nearly Always=4.

15. **Do you think that you do not have enough money to care for your relative, in addition to the rest of your expenses?**
Never =0; Rarely =1; Sometimes =2; Frequently =3, or Nearly Always=4.

16. **Do you think that you will be unable to take care of your relative much longer?**
Never =0; Rarely =1; Sometimes =2; Frequently =3, or Nearly Always=4.

17. **Do you think you have lost control of your life since your relative's illness?**
Never =0; Rarely =1; Sometimes =2; Frequently =3, or Nearly Always=4.

18. **Do you wish you could just leave the care of your relative to someone else?**
Never =0; Rarely =1; Sometimes =2; Frequently =3, or Nearly Always=4.

19. **Do you feel uncertain about what to do about your relative?**
Never =0; Rarely =1; Sometimes =2; Frequently =3, or Nearly Always=4.

20. **Do you think you could do a better job in caring for your relative?**
Never =0; Rarely =1; Sometimes =2; Frequently =3, or Nearly Always=4.

21. **Overall, how burdened do you think in caring for your relative?**
Never =0; Rarely =1; Sometimes =2; Frequently =3, or Nearly Always=4.

Total Score:_____

Scores of 41 or above indicate that a person may be experiencing caregiver burnout and a high degree of stress. If you scored in this range you need to discuss your thoughts and needs with a physician or seek caregiver support.

0 - 20 = little or no burden   **21 - 40 = mild to moderate burden**
41 - 60 = moderate to severe burden **61 - 88= severe burden**

Reference: Zarit SH, Reever KE, Bach-Peterson J. Relatives of the impaired elderly: correlates of feelings of burden. *Gerontologist*. 1980; 20(6):649-655.

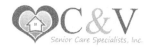

VALUE OF SUPPORT GROUPS

Sometimes you feel "stuck" – you have tried different approaches and nothing seems to work. You feel frustrated and you lose your ability to think creatively. This is where the power of the group makes an impact. You can draw on the support as well as the creativity of others in dealing with challenging behaviors.

The Alzheimer's Association sponsors support groups that serve as lifelines for many caregivers. Not only do these groups provide a place where you can meet other people who are living through the same type of struggles that you are experiencing, they provide education as well.

You learn that you are not alone; that others understand and accept your feelings of anger and frustration; and that you can talk freely and have your thoughts accepted. However you also learn from other caregivers as well as the group leader different strategies that have worked with other individuals with AD.

Check in your area to see if there are Memory Cafes. These are places where caregivers get together in a social situation that allows for sharing of experiences and feelings.

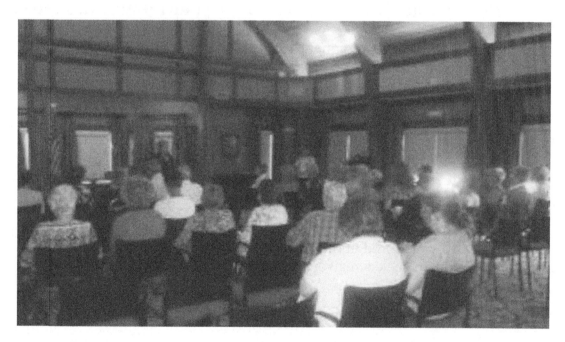

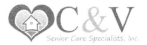

USING BEHAVIOR LOGS
The Value of Tracking the "Who, What and When" Behind Challenging Behaviors

Time	Activity	Behavior	People Around	Medication	Comment
Dementia Behavior Analysis					
7:00					
7:00					
7:30					
8:00					
8:30					
9:00					
9:30					
10:00					
10:30					
11:00					
11:30					
12 Noon					
12:30					
1:00					
1:30					
2:00					
2:30					
3:00					
3:30					
4:00					
4:30					
5:00					
5:30					
6:00					
6:30					
7:00					
7:30					
8:00					
8:30					
9:00					
9:30					
10:00					
10:30					
11:00					
11:30					
12 Midnight					
12:30					
1:00					
1:30					
2:00					
2:30					
3:00					
3:30					
4:00					
4:30					
5:00					
5:30					
6:00					
6:30					

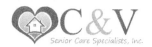

KEEPING GOOD RECORDS

It is important that you keep records of the behaviors of individual with AD; what you do in response to these behaviors; and how the person/your loved one responds to what you do. You are an expert on this person with AD. You know this person better than any other caregiver. Your observations may provide the key for other caregivers in knowing how to reach the individual. Your observations of what triggers a catastrophic reaction or an emotional outburst may assist in planning how to prevent a future catastrophic reaction or an emotional outburst. Pay attention to what words and actions calm and comfort the individual and what words and actions lead to distress. The focus of your observations is to keep the individual calm, peaceful and happy as much as possible and to keep your life under control as well.

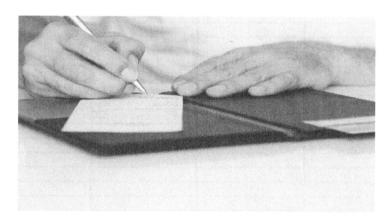

Not only is it important that you keep a record of the individual's behaviors, it is also important to keep a record of the individual's response to medications. The physician will appreciate your observations regarding whether or not a medication is making a positive impact on the targeted problem. For example, if the doctor adds a new medication to help the individual sleep better the doctor will want to know how many hours the individual is sleeping and if there are new problematic behaviors since starting the sleep medication such as falling or an increase in disorientation or confusion. You are the expert – help the professionals provide better care as a result of your observations and records.

It is also important to keep a readily accessible updated chart that lists important telephone numbers in case of an emergency. This is valuable to post within your home but also to carry with you.

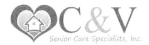

IMPORTANT NUMBERS AT A GLANCE

	Name	Phone Number	Fax Number	E-Mail
Caregiver				
Insurance Co.				
Secondary Insurance				
Primary Physician				
Physician's Assistant				
Office Manager				
Billing Department				
Doctor				
Office Manager				
Hospital				
Bank				
Relative				
Relative				
Alzheimer's Association				
Place of Worship				
Friend				
Attorney				
Accountant				

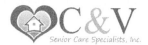

MEDICATION LOG

Name of Medicine	Dosage and frequency	Date Prescribed	Date Discontinued	Response to Drug

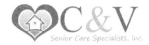

TAKING CARE OF YOU!

Staying Healthy While Coping with the Demands of Caregiving

The work of caregiving is incredibly challenging. It is important that you take care of yourself. It will do neither you nor your loved one any good if you get sick. There are things you need to do for yourself to maintain your physical, emotional, and spiritual health.

Physical Health:

- Make sure you get regular medical checkups and follow through with whatever your doctor suggests.
- It is important that you follow a healthy diet, exercise and get enough sleep.
- It is important that you give yourself a break-ask for help so you can get out of the house.
- Ask for family members to give you some time; inquire at your church to see if there are volunteers who could come in to stay with your loved one; if necessary pay someone to come in so you can get out.
- Explore respite services; look into whether your place of worship has a Faith Community Nurse.
- Arrange outdoor activities that include you and your loved one – take a walk together, go on short outings, go to church together.

Emotional Health:

- It is important to monitor your own moods, energy level, attitude, sleep and thoughts of optimism – you are at risk for depression – if you begin to feel low contact your physician, medication will help you cope.
- Talk to people about your sense of burden, how difficult and lonely your job is- talking won't make the job easier but it sure helps you to feel better about your situation.
- Seek out emotional support from your faith community, e.g. faith community nurse.
- Keep up activities and hobbies that give you pleasure- you need to continue to do things for you.
- Stay in contact with friends and family members – do not allow yourself to feel or become isolated.

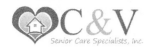

- Accept the fact that sometimes you feel really ANGRY, RESENTFUL, and TRAPPED- these thoughts are normal-admitting them actually makes it easier to deal with these thoughts in a positive manner.
- Find the joys in caregiving –there are joys – remember that you are doing a wonderful service by providing this care.

Spiritual Health

- It is important that you continue to do the activities that feed your spirit – pray, read Scripture, worship, sing- it is only out of a healthy and loving spirit that you can continue to provide care.
- Whatever activities that give your life meaning must be continued - you need to remain spiritually well.

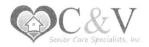

SECTION 2

UNDERSTANDING ALZHEIMER'S AND THE
THEORY OF RETROGENESIS

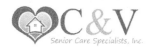

OVERVIEW OF ALZHEIMER'S DISEASE
AND RELATED DEMENTIAS

Alzheimer's disease is the number one Dementia – there are at least 100 different types of dementia but Alzheimer's makes up 65-70% of the dementias. Alzheimer's causes a steady decline in memory along with a loss of intellectual functions (thinking, remembering, and reasoning) serious enough to interfere with everyday life.

Some facts about Alzheimer's disease:

- It usually begins gradually

- The speed of the progression is very individual.

- It always causes confusion, personality and behavior changes, and impaired judgment.

- Communication becomes difficult until at the end of the disease the person has no "words" left to speak.

- It leads to total dependence.

What is the difference between Alzheimer's disease and normal age-memory difficulties?

Activity	A Person with Alzheimer's Disease	A Person with Age-Associated Memory Problems
Forgets	Whole experiences	Parts of an experience
Remembers later	Rarely	Often
Can follow written or spoken directions	Gradually unable	Usually able
Can use notes	Gradually unable	Usually able
Can care for self	Gradually unable	Usually able

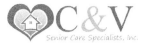

A TRIP THROUGH THE BRAIN: BRAIN DAMAGE LINKED TO SPECIFIC BEHAVIORS

Sometimes those with Alzheimer's are accused of "deliberately" saying or doing things to make the caregiver upset. Understanding that the challenging behaviors are directly linked to brain deterioration increases patience – at least a little!

It is important for caregivers to be able to link challenging behaviors with specific damage to the brain. When caregivers know and understand that the person's behaviors are not deliberate attempts to make the caregiver upset or angry, the behaviors are tolerated just a bit more. So often the person with Alzheimer's is unaware of the impact of his/her behaviors on the caregiver. So let's take our walk through the brain!

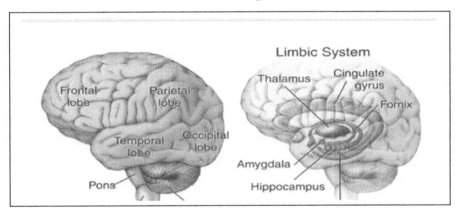

First hippocampus – stores short term memory; Middle stage, the hippocampus no longer functions – NO NEW LEARNING

Frontal Lobe- where we know what is appropriate-damage leads to inappropriate behaviors, cursing, and making hurtful comments to others.

Parietal lobes -where spatial processing is housed-problems in perception as well as in navigating first unfamiliar locations – later familiar locations.

Temporal lobes control time awareness and language- word finding problems –

Occipital lobe –can't identify things that are seen – misuse objects; trouble understanding and thinking very concrete

Motor Strip – controls walking, sitting up, continence and swallowing

Limbic system-emotional roller coaster

Hypothalamus – controls temperature and appetite

If you could see into the center of the brain through the temporal lobe you would be able to see where the hippocampus, the limbic system and the hypothalamus are located.

Amygdala-involved in processing emotions; linked to both fear and pleasure responses.

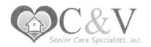

What does this mean?

The **Hippocampus** located deep in the brain processes every experience we have and saves them as short term memories. It saves the last 3-5 years of short term memories. One of the first symptoms that families and friends are aware of in someone with Alzheimer's is the repetition of questions or stories- because the person doesn't remember asking the questions or telling the story. In the middle stage, people only have about 5 minutes of short term memory – so if you say or do something that meets with a negative response you can walk away- return 5 minutes later and try a different approach-the person won't remember the first suggestion. This is sad for the person with Alzheimer's but a wonderful piece of information for the caregiver.

The **Hypothalamus** is located in the same area as the Hippocampus. The Hypothalamus controls appetite and body temperature. In the beginning of the middle stage – the Hypothalamus stops sending signals to indicate "fullness" even after eating a big meal. The person will repeat "When are we going to eat?" over and over again – because he/she not only doesn't remember eating (damage to the Hippocampus) but also because the Hypothalamus is not sending signals of fullness – what do you do? You provide finger foods and allow the individual to graze all day. At the end of the middle stage the Hypothalamus will not send signals of hunger so the person will not want to eat and can lose 20-30% of total body weight. One of the strategies to keep the person eating is to pour chocolate syrup, or jelly or something else sweet over the meal- many people retain their taste for sweets. The Hypothalamus also controls internal body temperature – most people with Alzheimer's complain of feeling cold at the end of the Middle stage of the disease – regardless of the ambient temperature.

The **Limbic System** is in the same area as the Hippocampus and Hypothalamus – we call this the "dementia neighborhood". The Limbic system controls emotions and explains why the person with Alzheimer's is on an emotional roller-coaster – quickly moving from sadness, to happiness and then to anger. It is not you that cause this - it is Alzheimer's and the damage it has done to the brain.

The **Parietal Lobe** controls the ability to get from one place to another. Initially people with Alzheimer's will get lost when traveling to unfamiliar locations but eventually will have trouble navigating in familiar locations.

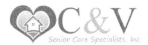

The **Motor Strip** controls the ability to go to the bathroom unaided, to remain continent and to handle the mechanics of toileting. It also controls the ability to walk, to sit up, and to swallow. Each of these skills becomes seriously impaired in the Middle stage of Alzheimer's. People become incontinent first of urine than of stool; they start to fall as their balance deteriorates; they have difficulty swallowing and may need to move to pureed foods and thickened liquids; by the end of the middle stage of the disease they are having increased difficulty sitting up.

Damage to the **Occipital Lobe** produces something called "visual agnosia". The person can still see the objects before him/her but no longer knows what/how that object is used. For instance, a person with Alzheimer's might pick up a television remote control and try to use it as a telephone, or pick up a tooth brush and attempt to brush her/his hair.

Damage to the **Temporal Lobes** interferes with the individual's time awareness and communication skills. By the end of the disease, if a person moves through all three stages of Alzheimer's, the person will lose the ability to speak.

Damage to the **Frontal Lobe** leads to inappropriate behavior- cursing, saying unkind and inappropriate comments.

Damage to the **Amygdala** in the Limbic system leads to difficulty processing emotions – excessive anger and fear can result from this damage.

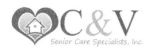

Mild Alzheimer's – "Great Foolers" Cognitive Function 12 to 8 years old **Stage 4 on FAST**	Mild Alzheimer's Cognitive Function 12 to 8 years old **Stage 4 on FAST**
Able to complete self-care tasks Able to communicate needs and converse Able to ask for help Able to structure ordinary daily routines Able to follow simple, verbal instructions Able to learn in situational specific arenas–if skill is valued Able to understand and play familiar games Able to ambulate independently and safely if no physical impairment Able to use highly familiar tools safety–may need supervision for quality of work and for unforeseen hazards	Forgetfulness/short-term memory loss may admit memory not good Impairment in judgment-makes bad decisions Difficulty with calculations, handling money, paying bills, balancing the check book (easily scammed by dishonest people who prey on those with Alzheimer's) Routine tasks take longer Lack of safety awareness-poor understanding of physical deficits Difficulty with familiar tasks such as cooking, Difficulty finding specific words Lack of spontaneity Less initiative Trouble understanding long explanations, use of new devices, or secondary effects of action Becomes anxious easily or may have a tendency to withdraw Increasing disorientation regarding time and place– may begin to get lost driving a car Social withdrawal or depression Mood/personality changes
Moderate Dementia Cognitive Function 7 to 5 years old **Stage 5 on FAST**	**Moderate Dementia** Cognitive Function 7 to 5 years old **Stage 5 on FAST**
Still remembers significant details about themselves and their family Still require no assistance with eating or using the toilet	Requires assistance in dressing self–has difficulty choosing appropriate attire for occasion and/or weather. May have difficulty in sequencing clothing Be unable to recall their own address or telephone number or the high school or college from which they graduated Become confused about where they are or what day it is Have trouble with less challenging mental arithmetic; such as counting backward from 40 by subtracting 4s or from 20 by 2s
Moderately Severe Dementia Toddlers Cognitive Function 5 to 3-2 years old Lasts 2-8 years **Stage 6a - 6e on FAST**	**Moderately Severe Dementia Toddlers** Needs full-time Supervision ONLY 5 MINUTES OF SHORT TERM MEMORY **Stage 6a - 6e on FAST**
Able to initiate familiar activity if supplies are available and in reach and they receiver verbal and tactile cues Able to tell stories from past Able to read words slowly out loud Able to follow slow simple instructions Able to speak in short sentences or phrases; able to make needs known Able to sort, stack objects and do repetitive behaviors Able to sing, move to music, count Able to ambulate if no physical disability Able to think and name objects (a toddler in an adult body)	Can't safely live alone Problems recognizing family and friends Problems organizing thoughts/logical thinking Repeats statements and/or movements Trouble dressing – may not want to bathe Increasing disorientation and forgetfulness Can't find words – unconsciously fills in the blanks Suspicious, teary, fidgety, irritable, silly Challenging behaviors apparent

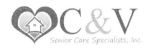

Stage 7 on FAST	
7a Speaks 5-6 words 7B single word—may repeat word over and over 7C Cannot walk without assistance 7D Cannot sit up without assistance Complete dependence Can smile at the beginning of the end stage Can swallow thickened liquids at the beginning of the end stage May put everything in mouth or touch everything	Cannot control bladder and bowel Increasing need for sleep Increasing difficulty swallowing Loses ability to walk and becomes bedridden Loses ability to sit up 7e Loses the ability to smile 7f Can no longer hold head up

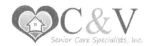

THEORY OF RETROGENESIS

Theory means "back to birth" or "back to the beginning". If you review the previous teaching tool on Stages of Alzheimer's you see that the stages correspond to:

Early Stage: Pre-adolescent deteriorating to the level of a 5 year old

Middle Stage: Toddler – 4 years of age deteriorating to the level of a 2 year old

End Stage: 18 month old deteriorating to newborn

Why is this theory so easy to understand and apply?

Because most of us have some experience with children. The application of this theory **DOES NOT ADVOCATE TREATING ADULTS WITH ALZHEIMER'S LIKE SMALL CHILDREN OR BABIES.** Then you might be asking how does knowing the cognitive and functional level help me manage my loved one's behaviors? Some of the same strategies that work with a child will also work with an adult who is cognitively and functionally behaving like a child.

A few examples will make this clear. Let's take a look at one of the challenging behaviors seen in those with Alzheimer's disease.

Repetition: Have you ever taken a trip with a young child- say a three year old, who asked repeatedly "Are we there yet mommy?" Or perhaps the child states, "I have to go potty." The strategies that parents use to respond to repetition in a toddler are similar to those that we use with an adult who repeats the same question or motion over and over again. We redirect the child. We sing songs with children; we engage them in a game that is repetitive; we give them snacks – we engage them in activities. These same strategies work equally well with adults with Alzheimer's disease. We might give the adult a repetitive activity to perform – the activity needs to be not only repetitive, but also productive and mindless. An activity that works well for many women is the activity of folding towels or other laundry or sweeping the floor. Men might sort coins; or nuts, bolts, and screws – all productive, mindless and repetitive activities. If you do this

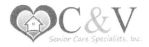

you are decreasing the repetition and redirecting the person into an acceptable activity!

Sometimes repetition requires a different approach – because the repetition may mean something other than, "I am bored." Repetition could mean the person is in pain, or is hungry or some other reason is driving the repetition. In those situations other responses are called for and we will discuss how to respond to the other reasons behind repetition when we talk about challenging behaviors.

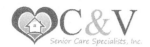

PHARMACOLOGICAL TREATMENT

While there is no cure for AD, there are drugs to treat the symptoms and retard the progression of the disease.

DRUG NAME	USED FOR	MANUFACTURER'S RECOMMENDED DOSAGE	COMMON SIDE EFFECTS
Namenda® (Memantine) Blocks the toxic effects of excess glutamine and regulates glutamine activation	Moderate to severe AD	5 mg once a day increase to 10 mg/day (5mg twice a day), 15 mg (5 mg and 10 mg as separate doses) and 20 mg/day (10 mg twice a day) at minimum of one week intervals if tolerated well	Dizziness, headache, constipation, confusion
Razadyne® (formerly known As Reminyl ® (galantamine) cholinesterase inhibitor*	Mild to Moderate AD	4 mg twice a day (8 mg/day) increase by 8 mg/day after 4 weeks to 16 mg/day if well tolerated; after another 4 weeks increase to 12 mg twice a day (24mg/day) if well tolerated	Nausea, vomiting, diarrhea, weight loss
Exelon® (rivastigmine) cholinesterase inhibitor*	Mild to Moderate AD	1.5 mg twice a day (3 mg/day) increase by 3 mg/day day every 2 weeks to 6mg twice a day (12 mg/day) if well tolerated	Nausea, vomiting, weight loss, upset stomach, muscle weakness
Aricept® (donepezil) cholinesterase inhibitor*	Mild to Moderate AD	5 once a day increase after 4-6 weeks to 10 mg once a day if well tolerated	Nausea, diarrhea, vomiting

*Cholinesterase inhibitors can increase the risk of stomach ulcers. Use NSAID's with caution in combination with these medications, since NSAID's can also cause stomach ulcers with prolonged use

Those with Alzheimer's may also be on a wide range of other medications for pain, for some challenging behaviors and for co-occurring medical diagnoses in addition to Alzheimer's.

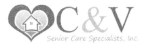

WHAT ARE POSSIBLE COMPLICATIONS OF ALZHEIMER'S DISEASE?

Pneumonia can happen if the individual has difficulty swallowing foods and liquids. If food or liquid gets into their lungs, the person with AD can develop pneumonia. It is important for caregivers to be aware of swallowing difficulties. These difficulties warrant the services of the Speech and Language Therapist.

Infections (like a urinary tract infection or UTI) can occur if the individual is incontinent and needs a catheter. This increases the risk of urinary infection. A UTI can occur just because the person doesn't drink enough – he/she doesn't ask for a drink – the caregiver needs to provide drinks on a regular (EVERY 2 HOURS) basis – and even more frequently when the outside temperature is hot.

Falls and their complications can be a real problem if the individual becomes more disoriented. Falls can lead to fractures and head injuries. Preventing falls is one of the jobs of the Physical Therapist.

What I should report to the Doctor or Nurse?

Report right away any of the following problems:

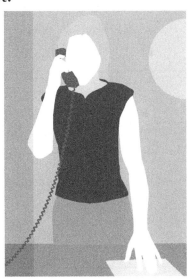

- Signs and symptoms of infection, especially respiratory or urinary tract: fever, cough and difficulty with urination;
- Any injury, especially injury from falls;
- Marked increase in confusion, hallucinations or aggressive behavior;
- Decreased food and fluid intake;
- Increased incontinence of bladder and bowel
- Weight loss of over 2 pounds in a week.
- Change in facial expression – sadness, withdrawing from others, not talking or taking part in family activities can all be signs of depression or some other physical problem that needs to be investigated.

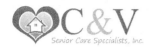

PERSISTENT SADNESS (DEPRESSION) AND ALZHEIMER'S DISEASE

Depression can be an added problem from the early stage of Alzheimer's disease through the middle stage. During the early stage the individual may be aware that he/she is losing something vitally important – they may know something is wrong. Depression is a common response to this awareness. However, depression can also occur in the middle stage of AD – Alzheimer's disease is stressful and stress depletes the chemicals needed to balance mood. Depression causes confusion, interferes with sleep and appetite so it is important that it be treated throughout the disease. Without treatment it will cause the dementia to appear worse than it is. Signs and symptoms of depression include:

- Sad face
- Change in appetite
- Change in weight
- Change in sleep patterns
- Slow movements
- Crying
- Expressions of despair and hopelessness
- Suicidal thinking

Depression in Alzheimer's disease needs to be treated with one of the antidepressants. It is important to share your observations of the individual's depressed behavior with the nurse and/or physician.

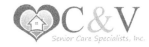

RECOGNIZING PAIN AND DEALING WITH IT

Pain is frequently unrecognized and therefore not treated in those with Alzheimer's disease. Let's apply the Theory of Retrogenesis to understand this situation.

This is the scenario: Imagine you are taking care of a toddler – a child between 2 and 4 years of age. The child seems "out of sorts" and fussy. You notice that the child lacks energy, he is not interested in eating and his

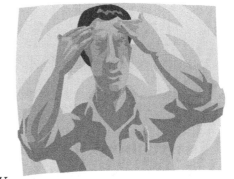

color seems a bit "off" – perhaps he looks pale and you notice that he occasionally pulls on his ear. He is not interested in playing and "mops" around. At night time he sleeps fitfully, frequently calling out to you – thus interfering with your sleep. In the morning you call the pediatrician to report what you have concluded is an ear infection. Not once has this little boy said, "Mommy my ear hurts." Or "Please give me a Baby Tylenol for my ear-ache." Or even "Can I have some of that pink medicine you gave me the last time my ear hurt?" The child says none of these things but parents, grandparents and other caregivers to the very young are attuned to the changes in behavior that indicate there is something physically wrong! The primary caregiver may call the pediatrician and say, "Johnny isn't eating or drinking, he didn't sleep last night and I noticed that he has been pulling on his ear. I think he might have another ear infection."

This same knowledge needs to be applied to the person with Alzheimer's, who is in the middle or late stage of the disease and is functioning at the level of a toddler or younger. This person does not have the ability to say, "My joints hurt," or, "when I pee it hurts me", or "I have a headache." The caregiver must be attuned to these non-verbal ways that the person is communicating PAIN. All too often the caregiver of an Alzheimer's individual interprets restlessness, problems sleeping, lack of appetite, and aggression during bathing, dressing and other activities of daily living as psychotic and/or anxious behaviors. Because the caregiver fails to recognize pain, the caregiver calls the primary or attending physician if the person is living in an Assisted Living Facility or in a Skilled Nursing Facility and requests either anxiety medication or antipsychotic medication – neither of which will address the issue of pain – but what they will do is decrease the ability of the person to communicate the pain!

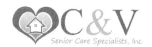

The following tool, developed for children, is a wonderful tool to assess both **pain** and **depression** in those with Alzheimer's disease.

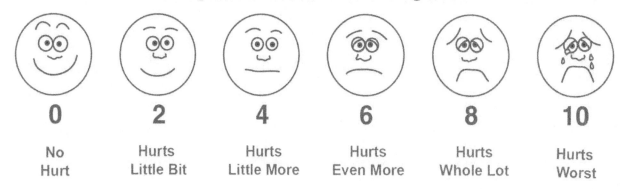

Wong-Baker FACES® Pain Rating Scale

0	2	4	6	8	10
No Hurt	Hurts Little Bit	Hurts Little More	Hurts Even More	Hurts Whole Lot	Hurts Worst

www.wongbakerFACES.org   ©1983 Wong-Baker FACES® Foundation. Used with permission.

Instructions for Usage: Explain to the person that each face is for a person who has no pain (hurt) or some, or a lot of pain.

Face 0 doesn't hurt at all. Face 2 hurts just a little bit. Face 4 hurts a little bit more. Face 6 hurts even more. Face 8 hurts a whole lot. Face 10 hurts as much as you can imagine, although you don't have to be crying to have this worst pain.

Ask the person to choose the face that best depicts the pain they are experiencing.

IT IS IMPERATIVE THAT CAREGIVERS OF THOSE WITH ALZHEIMER'S RECOGNIZE PAIN AND NOT CONFUSE PAIN WITH ANXIOUS OR PSYCHOTIC BHAVIOR.

The same faces can be used to assess for sadness and depression

Face "0" = **Very Happy**
Face "2" = **Happy**
Face "4" = **Not Sad, Not Happy**
Face "6" = **Sad**
Face "8" = **Sad Most of the Time**
Face "10" = **Sad All of the Time**

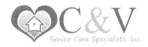

HOME SAFETY ASSESSMENT

YES	NO	N/A	GENERAL:	YES	NO	N/A	BATHROOM
☐	☐	☐	1. Are medications safely and adequately labeled?	☐	☐	☐	27. Does the bathroom have a non-skid surface?
☐	☐	☐	2. Are guns or weapons safely stored?	☐	☐	☐	28. Are there adequately placed grab bars (not towel bars) in the bathroom? (by toilet, in shower).
☐	☐	☐	3. Are throw rugs, area rugs, and flooring materials secured?	☐	☐	☐	
☐	☐	☐	4. Is there adequate lighting in each room?				29. If precautions necessitate, is there a properly installed raised toilet seat?
☐	☐	☐	5. Are there telephone cords or electrical cords in walkway?	☐	☐	☐	
☐	☐	☐	6. Are there outlets with too many plugs?				30. Is there an adequate shower/tub bench present?
☐	☐	☐	7. Are combustibles, such as newspapers, stored at least three feet from stove, fireplace or heaters?	☐	☐	☐	31. Is water heater set at 120° or lower?
☐	☐	☐	8. Is there adequate space around space heaters?				**Comments:**
☐	☐	☐	9. Are there exposed heating pipes?				
☐	☐	☐	10. Is the room/house heated/cooled adequately and safely?	☐	☐	☐	**KITCHEN**
☐	☐	☐	11. Is the water in the kitchen, bathroom, and utility area working properly in each room?	☐	☐	☐	32. Are commonly used items stored for safe and easy access?
☐	☐	☐	12. Do the entry doors lock with deadbolts?	☐	☐	☐	33. Do the stove and/or microwave operate properly?
☐	☐	☐	13. Are emergency phone numbers easily readable and visible and are occupants able to summon help?	☐	☐	☐	34. Is there a portable fire extinguisher available in the kitchen?
☐	☐	☐	14. Do occupants who are smokers demonstrate safe handling of cigarettes, lighters and matches?	☐	☐	☐	35. Are all occupants who have the opportunity to cook able to safely operate kitchen appliances, use knives and work with fire?
☐	☐	☐	15. Does the gas at the stove, furnace, space heater work properly?				
☐	☐	☐	16. Are walkways clear, sturdy and wide enough to walk safely (using assistive devices if necessary)?	☐	☐	☐	36. Is there adequate refrigeration?
☐	☐	☐					**Comments:**

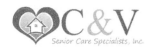

☐	☐	☐	17. If burglar bars are present on doors and/or windows, will they bend for emergency exit or is the key close by?	☐	☐	☐	**ACTIVITIES OF DAILY LIVING (ADL'S)**
☐	☐	☐	18. Is there a phone in easy reach?	☐	☐	☐	37. Do all assistive devices for ambulation fit the owner properly?
☐	☐	☐	19. Is there a working smoke detector near the kitchen and near each sleeping area?	☐	☐	☐	38. Are all required assistive devices and medical equipment used properly?
☐	☐	☐	20. Are there signs of rodent or pest infestation?				
☐	☐	☐	21. If oxygen is in use in the house, are all occupants aware of oxygen and cord safety?	☐	☐	☐	39. Are all required ADL assistive devices present and in good working order?
☐	☐	☐	22. Are all occupants able to safely exit the home in five minutes or less?	☐	☐	☐	40. Does individual have enough endurance to perform basic self-care?
☐	☐	☐	23. Have arrangements been made to remove snow and ice from steps and driveways? 24. Are there secure handrails on stairs? 25. Are hazardous materials stored safely? 26. If a ramp is needed, is one present and safely constructed?

Comments: | ☐ | ☐ | ☐ | 41. Does individual require energy conservation, work simplification, or graded endurance training? 42. If a wheelchair is used in the house, are doorways wide enough for safe operation of the wheelchair? 43. If transfer assistance is required by a individual, are these transfers performed safely? **Comments:** |

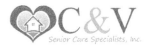

LIFE STORY

My name is: _____. I like to be called: _____
My birthday is_____. I was born in
(city/state)_____

My family members are (names of parents and sisters and brothers)

My memories of my school days: (what schools? Years attended? Powerful memories of school, friends, teachers?)

My jobs included:

I am/was married to: _____for _____years.
I was never married/divorced but the most important people in my life are:

I have children and their names are:

I have grandchildren and their names are:

I enjoyed (interests, hobbies, events):

I have always enjoyed talking about:

I am/am not a religious person. My faith community is_____

When I look back over my life, I am most proud of:

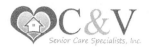

When I look back over my life some of my most powerful memories are:

I love/don't love pets.
My favorite pet is/was a _____ named_____

These are some of the things I do/have done frequently (walk the dog, read the morning/evening paper, watch television news, watch sports, garden, cook, get together with family/friends, shower in the morning, say my prayers, read Scripture):

My favorite music is:

I love to/don't' love to dance.
I have always been/have not been physically active.

Other things that make me special and unique include:

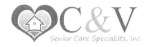

SECTION 3

COMMUNICATING WITH SOMEONE WITH ALZHEIMER'S DISEASE

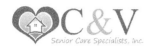

16 BASIC STRATEGIES FOR COMMUNICATING WITH THE ALZHEIMER'S INDIVIDUAL/LOVED ONE

Keep it Simple – it's the rule when communicating with a loved one with memory loss. Here are some helpful tips:

1. Easy as 1-2-3

Say the individual's name and identify yourself to him or her **even if you are a family member this includes everyone - adult children, grandchildren and even the spouse. If the person has forgotten the relationship – reminding him/her that you are the "daughter" or "spouse" might only upset him/her – just saying for example, "Hi John, I am Sherrie, and I came to visit with you today." As opposed to "Hi Dad – I am here to see you today."**

2. The speaker must be willing to enter the person's world. For instance, if the person tells you that he/she just went to a Yankees game (and that is not reality) – you ask about the game – Who won? Did you have a good time? Did you eat a hotdog? Tell me all about it.

3. Keep it positive (avoid the negative)

> ➤ Negative: "Don't put your hand in the gravy".
> ➤ Positive: "Please put your hands in your lap" (use gestures).

4. How to handle choices

"We are having macaroni for lunch today." (smile) versus "What would you like for lunch today?" There are exceptions. Remember life is about daily change. Be flexible. If you need to ask a question, limit the choices given. "Would you like chicken or macaroni today?"

5. Keep it simple

Simplify your statements-avoid being lengthy. The person with Alzheimer's may forget the first part of the explanation before the speaker is even finished!

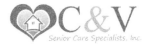

6. One step at a time
Break tasks into simple steps:
"Pick up the comb."
"Comb your hair."
"Pick up your toothbrush."
"Put the toothbrush on your teeth."
"Move the toothbrush etc.

7. Speak to your loved one as an adult
Be aware of your tone of voice. Remember to preserve your loved one's dignity at all times. It is common to use the word "we" as in "Don't we look pretty today? Instead, say "You look very nice today." This is more respectful.

8. Non-Verbal Communication
Tone of voice, facial expressions, touch and gestures are effective and important parts of communicating with your loved one.

Tone of voice
Listen to your own tone of voice; it speaks volumes. The person with memory loss maintains the ability to understand tone of voice, even after the ability to understand words has been lost. Listen to your loved ones' tone of voice; it will reveal her/his message more so than his/her words.

Facial expression
Know that your loved one is able to read your facial expressions even though you may not even be aware of them. When we speak to someone we usually look them in the eye to assess their feelings or their intentions. The entire face-eyes, forehead, nose, eyebrows and cheeks-communicate a vast range of emotions to others. We are able to convey happiness, fear, anger, disgust, surprise, remorse and sadness. Be aware when speaking with your loved one as well as with others, that your facial expressions speak a thousand words.

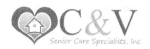

Touch

It is important to offer your loved one reassurance. Hugs work wonders. Touching someone's arm or shoulder, holding their hand, patting their back; all of these forms of touch provide comfort and pleasure. Be aware of moving someone in their wheelchair without letting them know first, with a gentle touch and reminder, 'need to move you to the table now." Pulling someone in their chair in An abrupt manner is very insensitive. Provide a gentle touch and you will bring a smile to your loved one's heart.

Gestures

We use gestures daily to communicate our needs-hand gestures to describe how large something is, pointing in the correct direction to guide someone, waving to say "hello." Using simple gestures is helpful as a complementary addition to your words and your tone of voice. Remember to avoid gestures that could be misinterpreted as threatening to your loved one.

9. Speak slowly

It takes longer for a person with memory loss to process what was said. By speaking calmly and slowly, you have a much greater chance of being understood.

10. Be aware of hearing or vision problems

Older people suffer with these losses and it is important to remember they do not hear or see as well as we do. Have you ever smeared suntan oil on your sunglasses while at the beach? Imagine going through life daily with cloudy lenses, which is literally how some elders see.

11. Smile and the world smiles with you

If you look for the good and the positive in people and in life, you will find abundant opportunities to smile. Laughter is the best medicine, so use your sense of humor. Be sensitive **not to laugh at** your loved one, but at the situation.

12. Put logic and reason "on the shelf"

Confrontation with your loved one will only increase his/her level of agitation and anxiety. Instead of: "You know you're not supposed to wear that bra outside of your dress." Try suggesting: "Let me help you with this."

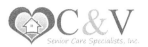

13. Remember to forget the phrase "don't you remember?"

Pretend your computerized brain has a glitch when it wants to say that phrase and erase it from your memory bank! "This is your daughter, Susan." Vs. "Don't you remember me? This approach helps the person "save face".

14. Always validate feelings

Even if the content of what your loved one is saying is "not real," the feelings are always real. An example of validating is "I know how upset you must be to think I'd steal your purse."

15. Use Signage:

Throughout the early and middle stages of Alzheimer's people can still read. Reading is an "old" skill – learned in the primary grades and reinforced every year that the person remained in school so it is an "over learned" skill. Whereas the spoken word literally goes in one ear and out the other, writing can stay in front of someone and be retained. Knowing that people can still read provides another strategy to deal with repetitive questions – you write the answer on a notepad and refer the person with Alzheimer's to the notepad!

16. Truthfulness may not always be the kindest response.

As the person loses memories he/she can no longer enter into your reality. Confronting that person with a reality such as the death of a loved one may actually be cruel. Forcing a person with a severe memory problem to hear a "truth" will cause emotional pain. It is better to validate the feelings the person is expressing rather than make her/him face a reality that is totally gone from memory.

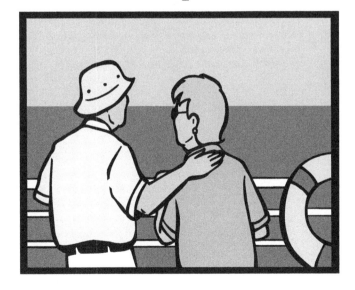

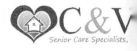

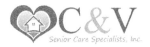

SECTION 4

MANAGING ACTIVITIES OF DAILY LIVING AND PHYSICAL CARE

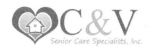

MAINTAINING AND INCREASING ORIENTATION

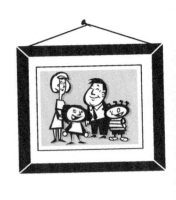

1. Use large calendars and clocks in easy to see locations
2. Decorate with seasonal items
3. Use chalk boards to write reminders
4. Have pictures of family on display
5. Create and use a "memory book"
6. Use memory aids such as making a list of the day's activities, phone numbers that can be called for help or writing out instructions for tasks like making a cup of tea. Label the contents of drawers.
7. Place arrows, signs, and pictures (i.e. picture of toilet on bathroom door) throughout house to assist person to independently get around.
8. The use of signage is an important tool – people can read well into the disease – so using signs to remind them to use the bathroom, to inform them what drawers hold underwear and socks, to encourage the use of a walker, and to provide the answer to a repetitive question such as "Where are we going?" - the use of signs keeps the caregiver calm and the person with Alzheimer's disease more independent.
9. Establish regular times for eating, exercising, bathing, outings, etc.
10. Remember that "routine is a substitute for memory" – try to maintain "sameness" in as many activities as possible.
11. Maintain "sameness" in home – don't rearrange furniture unless arrangement poses a safety risk.....
12. Limit choices
13. Avoid clutter
14. Avoid over-stimulation
15. Avoid under-stimulation
16. Use clothing that is easy off and on
17. Install adequate lighting
18. Install locks on doors – out of line of vision – very high or very low on door.
19. Install child-proof door openers on closet doors that might be used to store cleaning supplies – otherwise keep these supplies locked up
20. Identify the proper bedroom by placing a picture of your loved one on the door.
21. Get in the habit of saying, "It is Monday and today we ...."; "It is dinner time"; "It is time to take a walk." Structure the routine for both you as the caregiver and your loved one.

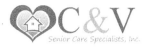

WAYS TO MAINTAIN INDEPENDENCE

1. Use of raised and contrasting color toilet seat.

2. Use of hand-held shower.

3. Use of clothing that is easy to get on and off – pants with elastic waists, pull-over tops, Velcro instead of snaps.

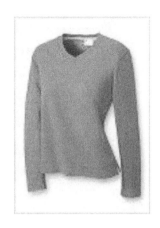

4. Use tennis shoes with Velcro closures instead of "shoe strings.

5. Use of grab bars.

6. Use of written instructions in large print

7. Avoid taking over activities for the person with Alzheimer's disease – encourage the continuation of activities of daily living even if these take longer or are messier (feeding self).

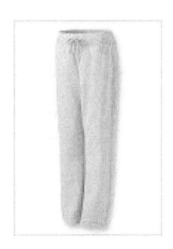

8. Use Signage – see previous tool.

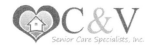

LIFE IS UNCERTAIN: EAT DESSERT FIRST!

Most of the time we are concerned with people eating the recommended number of servings from the food pyramid. For those with Alzheimer's, our concern shifts to making sure that they don't lose weight. Losing weight puts them at great risk for skin breakdown, infections, falls and other complications. Three square meals a day with afternoon and evening snacks just doesn't cut it with this individual. We need to change our thinking – it is okay to eat dessert first!

How should we approach the person with Alzheimer's or another Dementia?

1.   As an individual – what is the person's favorite foods? He/she can have as much of that food as he/she wants!

2.   When does the person want to eat? The individual may prefer to get up late and is a "night owl" and likes eating little bits at a time, but all day long!

3.   What if the person repeats over and over again, even after eating a large meal, "when are we going to eat? We allow him/her to eat "finger food" – pieces of fruit, cheese, cracker and other snacks. Complaints of hunger mean that the Hypothalamus in the brain is no longer sending them signals of fullness – this usually happens at the beginning of the middle stage. At the end of the middle stage the Hypothalamus will stop sending signals of hunger so the person will not want to eat and can lose 20-30% of her total body weight. At that point we try to counter this by making the food sweet – pouring maple syrup or chocolate syrup over the food frequently encourages the person to continue to eat. The food may also have to be pureed towards the end of the disease because of swallowing difficulties.

What do we need to do?

1.   Serve major caloric meal early in the day – possible to start day with a really hearty breakfast – eggs, meat, pancakes, and other well-liked breakfast foods – don't forget the condiments – lots of butter and syrup. Lunch should be a mid-size meal with soup, salad and a sandwich. Dinner time should be a one utensil meal – pizza and salad; sandwich and cookies.

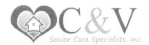

2. Serve meal on brightly colored dinnerware – a color contrast between the tablecloth or placemat and the dinnerware serves as a visual cue for self-feeding.

3. Offer courses one at a time with only the needed utensils to not overwhelm the individual. Place beverages directly in front of the person and not off to the side.

4. Prevent spills by filling cups only half full.

5. Assure good dental health – broken, decayed teeth may cause pain that interferes with eating; make sure to provide mouth care after a meal to make sure that the individual is not pocketing the food, which is an indicator of impaired swallowing.

6. Need to promote snacking whenever the individual is awake.

7. Provide foods that are calorie dense and dementia friendly – peanut butter sandwiches; milkshakes with an added protein supplement; pudding cups; ice cream, pureed fruit, and sweetened yogurt.

8. Don't be upset if your loved one wants to eat his roast beef and mashed potatoes with sugar sprinkled on top.

9. Keep lots of drinks available – juice, soda, water, decaffeinated tea – be constant in your encouragement drink – offer something to drink every 2 hours while the person is awake. Just like a toddler the person in the middle stage of Alzheimer's will not ask for drinks. The caregiver needs to anticipate this need and offer drinks throughout the day. This will also help to prevent urinary tract infections.

10. Use finger foods when possible. Pre-cut food into small pieces, avoid stringy or hard to chew foods.

11. Provide hand-over-hand assistance for the person to begin using a utensil.

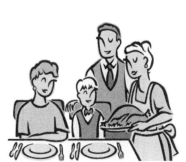

12. Eat with your loved one and offer encouragement and praise throughout the meal.

13. Choose foods with strong flavors hot or cold instead of tepid to add to appeal.

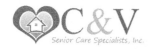

14.   Individual should be in sitting position to facilitate swallowing and to prevent choking.

15.   Decrease distractions and make surroundings pleasant and calming. Feed individual as soon as he/she is seated and turn off the TV.

16.   Enrich foods with fortified milk (powdered milk mixed with whole milk).

17.   Offer liquid supplement to increase calories – instant breakfast drinks mixed with ice cream are often more appealing than commercial products.

18.   Provide personal assistance to the individual.

19.   Limit "dining out" experiences – the choices, the unfamiliarity of the dining area, music, mirrors, chairs with wheels, and crowds can all add up to an over stimulating environment and lead to a sudden behavior decline.

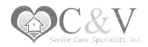

HOW DO WE MANAGE THE PERSON'S DIFFICULTY WITH SWALLOWING?

1. Stimulate the mouth to open by brushing the spoon against the lips.

2. Place food well into mouth.

3. Give only small amounts of food at one time.

4. Give frequent reminders of the expected behavior (e.g. say, "Open your mouth, chew the food, and now swallow) because individuals can forget that they are eating.

5. Gently brush the cheeks and neck to encourage swallowing.

6. As soon as the individual swallows have the next bite of food ready.

7. Foods can be ground or pureed in a blender or baby food grinder.

8. Thin liquids are the most difficult to swallow.
   - Use a "sipping" cup with a lid or a "nosey" cup, which has a cut-out space to keep the cup from bumping into the nose.
   - Cold drinks are often easier to swallow than hot drinks.
   - Thickening agents can be purchased at most drug or discount stores.

9. Excessive drooling, pocketing of food, chocking, coughing, or a "gravelly" voice after eating may indicate the need for other swallowing strategies. The Speech-Language Pathologist can help you to learn how to facilitate safe swallowing in your loved one.

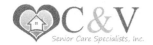

ENCOURAGING ADEQUATE HYDRATION AND PREVENTING URINARY INFECTIONS

It is really important for people with Alzheimer's Dementia to take in enough fluid. Without enough fluid the person's skin becomes dry and fragile and more prone to skin breakdown. Without enough fluid, urine becomes concentrated and the person is more prone to urinary infections. Without enough fluid, the person may become constipated and even impacted. None of these are good things!

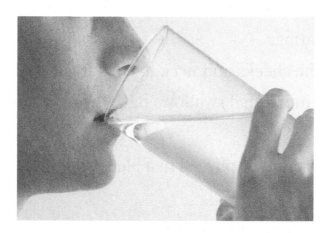

As the disease progresses, individuals with AD may not recognize that they are thirsty. We can't depend on the individual to take care of his own fluid needs nor can we expect that he/she will tell us that she/he is thirsty. It becomes essential that fluid intake is planned into the schedule of the day. Every hour or so the person with Alzheimer's should be offered something to drink and encouraged to drink as much as he/she wants. The offerings can be varied and include the individual's favorites. Does he like tea, coffee, cold water with a sliver of lemon, soda, milkshake, and/or juice? If you are able to provide a liquid that also supplies calories, such as juice or milkshake you can "kill two birds with one stone" so to speak! It is possible to maintain hydration as well as weight at the same time.

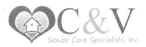

DEALING WITH INCONTINENCE
TIMED AND PROMPTED VOIDING SCHEDULES
First a Story from Beverly Bigtree Murphy to Help with Incontinence Management

Moments of Love during Trying Times

"He became completely incontinent by 1990. We were lucky again. The level of intimacy the two of us enjoyed with each other allowed an easier transition for us as his needs changed. The crossing point for both of us occurred when I realized he wasn't cleaning himself properly. I took the practical approach and offered what I saw as the only alternatives. Either he let me help, or someone else was going to have to help, or he'd end up dying of filth. Tom was pragmatic as always. As for my attitude towards doing 'it', I could see only four choices. I could choose anger, disgust, benign complacency, or love. I made the conscious effort to choose love. Assuring him I could also do this for him without revulsion or personal pain made the transition a lot easier for him and for me. Just to demonstrate that moments of tenderness were possible in what had to be thought of as an impossible breeding ground for such moments, I'll never forget the following incident...

Tom had contracted a stomach virus which brought with it all the horror one can only imagine in the care of someone with the combination of motor control and reasoning problems Tom had. If there is hell on earth, diarrhea in a late stage Alzheimer's person is it. If there is a heaven, it only lasts 24 hours. Given my state of sleep deprivation and the physical energy it took to handle Tom's relentless need for help, I was at my wits end as we once more made the trip to the bathroom with pajamas that had to be changed and floors that had to be cleaned. I wanted to scream I felt so tired, and used, and spent, and unappreciated. And poor Tom, he was just responding to being sick and anxious from all the activity surrounding that night, getting more and more combative as the night wore on and as my own anxiety level increased. I remember steering him one more time into the bathroom and out of desperation, (I don't where the words came from), I uttered...

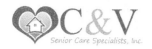

"Thank you, Lord!"

And Tom responded...

"Thank you for what?"

"It could be worse, Tom."

"How?"

"I might not still love you as much as I do."

He turned his head towards me and said...

"You still love me?"

"Of course, I love you."

"God, I love you too." I saw tears form in his eyes and he continued...

"Bevy!"

"What, Tom."

"Thank you."

The evening became one of sharing the absurdity of what was going on in our lives and one of reconnecting to each other. And it was a sort of turning point for me. I stopped thinking victimized by what Tom's care needs meant by simply moving out of anger and into love, realizing in the process that it was as easy as making the choice to do so. I had two choices in attending to Tom's needs and that was to do them happily or do them mad. Either way, they still had to be done. And I realized something else. I realized how much Tom still needed to be loved. After all, what were we actually dealing with? A little poop between lovers wasn't really that much of a big deal."

Used with permission of Beverly Bigmurphy.com *Moments of Love during Trying Times*, Accessed May 1st, 2014, http://bigtreemurphy.com/Using%20Usual%20Things.htm *Permission granted June 2014.*

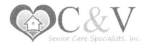

We opened this section with an excerpt from a phenomenal website, bigtreemuphy.com. Within this website you can find every detail that you might need to handle incontinence. Beverly Bigtree Murphy generously shares with readers the struggles and more importantly the successful strategies that she learned as she provided care for her husband Tom. Many of the strategies we suggest are taken from Beverly Bigtree Murphy's website.

Eventually everyone who is diagnosed with Alzheimer's disease will become incontinent. First the person becomes incontinent of urine than of stool. There is nothing you can do to prevent incontinence but lots that you can do to manage it! Some will advise you that incontinence is a reason for placement. This is not true. In fact many people with Alzheimer's start to have problems with incontinence while they are still pretty involved in the world- experiencing "accidents" in the early stage. Incontinence is not a reason for institutionalization - the caregiver can manage this and can develop the skills needed to keep her/his loved one home as long as that is a feasible option.

"Accidents" will happen before the person is totally incontinent. It is important to be a hovering presence – avoid discussions, reasoning and the details of your tasks to a minimum. During the daytime it helps to encourage the person to use the bathroom about every 2 hours but that is not always possible – so again the use of incontinence products are your safety net when you can't stick to a strict schedule. If the schedule adds to your stress than ignore it – just make sure you offer drinks frequently – otherwise you will be dealing with fecal impactions and urinary tract infections – better to avoid them if possible.

Do not ask the person if she/he needs help – most likely the person will say "no".

Work from behind the person – this minimizes your presence.

Treat incontinence pads in a matter of fact way just as if they are simply another part of the dressing routine. Avoid making statements like' It's time to change your diaper." Instead, use terms such as "showering", "bathing", "getting freshened up", or "getting ready for bed".

Do not ask for permission to use incontinence pads – this is your decision.

Have all the supplies needed to "clean someone" at hand and organized. You want to work efficiently, competently and matter of factly. Leave the cleaning up of the room until after the person is dressed and in another area.

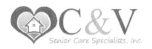

So let's take a look at some additional strategies that you can use:

1. Stock up on inexpensive washcloths sold in packages of 6 or 12. They are thin and allow the caregiver to get adequately clean the individual's bottom and grab hold of feces. Use different colors of the clothes for different functions – one color for incontinence care. Baby wipes and similar products are not only expensive but they don't provide a good grip, which is important when removing feces. Have a stack of these cloths ready –some soaped and some ready to rinse. If using the packaged products, which offer convenience on the road, pull them out before cleansing the person. Some of these are flushable. If traveling look for highway gas stations which offer more privacy of a single stall plus access to a sink. Always travel with a dispenser of liquid soap for cleansing – using a mixture of ½ soap and ½ water for ease in dispensing and at the same time doesn't put on too much soap. Use a dispenser with a pull top – tab tops get in the way.

2. To deal with "diaper rash" that can quickly escalate without proper treatment – use cold pressed castor oil or bag balm – both make good lubricants and salves for skin breakdown, rashes, etc.

3. Encourage your loved one to use the bathroom before bedtime. Do not awaken that person during the night to use the bathroom – not only will you be interfering with her/his sleep but yours as well. One of the major enemies to successful caregiving is the exhaustion of the caregiver – namely you!

Making the Bathroom a Safer and Friendlier Place for those with Alzheimer's – these suggestions are important for managing urinating and defecating but also bathing and brushing teeth as well.

1. Cover or remove wall to wall mirrors – seeing the reflections in the mirror confuses the person with AD who might have trouble determining whether there are strangers in the room – this may precipitate a catastrophic reaction where the person with AD and/or the caregiver gets hurt. Mirrors that are on a medicine cabinet do not generate the same response.

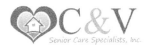

2. Change knobs, which are associated with burns, to handles on sinks and tubs.

3. Remove glass sliding doors – they are dangerous. It is better to replace with a shower curtain with metal grommets attached to a sturdy shower rod.

4. Additional supplies you will need – a hand held shower nozzle at least 7 feet long and a shower chair. When the person is no longer able to move under the shower head to rinse off they are probably afraid of the shower at that point (see our teaching tool on bathing and the value of the tootsie roll pop). This is when the hand held shower nozzle will work wonders in allowing you to thoroughly rinse the person.

5. Get rid of anything that is not absolutely necessary from the bathroom. Paint the walls a solid and soothing color. There should be few distractions on the walls or on flat surfaces – these changes help to decrease agitated and aggressive behaviors.

   When traveling by car it is better to handle incontinence issues in gas station bathrooms rather than large multi-stall bathrooms designed for either women or men – but not both. The bathroom in a service station is usually one room with a toilet and a sink – this allows the activities involved in cleaning someone's bottom to be done privately.

   Used with permission of Beverly Bigmurphy.com *Moments of Love during Trying Times, Accessed May 1st, 2014,* *http://bigtreemurphy.com/Using%20Usual%20Things.htm* *Permission granted June 2014.*

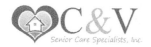

SKIN CARE TO PREVENT PRESSURE ULCERS

People with Alzheimer's disease are often at risk for pressure ulcers (bedsores) due to factors such as decreased activity, poor health, poor nutrition, confusion and/or lack of bladder or bowel control (incontinence). Ideally you want to prevent pressure ulcers – by encouraging enough liquid and a healthy diet and by making sure the position of a bed bound person is moved very two hours. Sometimes it is all most impossible to get a person with Alzheimer's disease who is in the last stage to take in adequate calories or fluid and maybe unable to independently move from side to side to take the pressure off of vulnerable pressure points on the body. If you have not engaged outside help either through certified (Medicare covered) or private duty home care – now might be the time to seek out this support.

What are Pressure Ulcers?

A pressure ulcer is an area of skin where lack of blood flow has caused tissue damage. Pressure ulcers can be caused if the bone presses on the skin while a person is sitting or lying for a long time or by the pressure of clothing or a shoe that is too tight.

Symptoms of Pressure Ulcers

The symptoms of pressure ulcers depend on the amount of damage to skin and tissue. Pressure ulcers are rated as follows:

- Stage I– redness of the skin; skin is not broken. In light-skinned people, a Stage 1 sore may change skin color to a dark purple or red area that does not become pale when pressed. In dark-skinned people, this area may become darker than normal.
- Stage II – blister or superficial break in the skin. Skin damage to the outer layer of skin, the epidermis, or the next layer, the dermis.
- Stage III – deep wound involving damage of tissue below the dermis into the subcutaneous layer (under the skin).
- Stage IV – deep would with damage to muscle or bone.

Who Is At Risk For Pressure Ulcers?

- People who are bed-bound or chair-bound
- People with poor circulation
- Those with a decreased sense of pain.
- People who are unable to control their urine flow or bowel movements
- People who are thin or frail
- People who are confused or in a coma

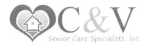

BATHING AND THE VALUE OF A TOOTSIE ROLL POP!

Bathing is an intimate experience; the person with dementia may find the bathing experience, frightening, embarrassing, or painful and may exhibit behaviors to express those thoughts such as resisting, screaming, and even hitting. The behaviors occur because the person does not clearly understand the purpose of bathing and may react to unpleasant aspects such as lack of modesty, thinking cold, water hitting her/his face and causing great fear or experiencing discomfort and because the caregiver does not understand the implications of the person's cognitive and functional age – probably that of a toddler. Bathing is the #1 activity that gets caregivers hit, bit, kicked and in a variety ways hurt!

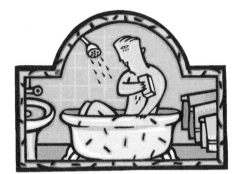

Resistance to bathing begins in the middle stage of AD when the person has a cognitive age of about 3 years of age. This is important to remember when the person gets upset with bathing – ask yourself – would a three year old get upset with the manner in which I am bathing this person with AD? If the answer is yes –then you need to find another strategy! To be more specific we do not generally shower toddlers. This is an area where application of the Theory of Retrogenesis can have dramatic implications. The water hitting the person in the face might be terrifying! Aren't there other ways to clean someone?

Try the following:

♦ **Do everything you can in advance to make the process easier,** such as increasing the temperature of the room (a cold room might aggravate joint pain if the person being bathed has arthritis), reduce overhead lighting, have bath towels and if possible, a terry cloth robe nearby. Provide familiar soap (the type and brand the individual has used in the past) and test the temperature of the water. Have a supply of "tootsie roll pops©" on hand or any other distracter that you think might work with the person to be bathed. Remember the person with Alzheimer's can only do one thing at a time and if it is something he/she enjoys like sucking on a tootsie roll – the caregiver can do just about anything else that needs

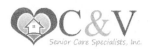

to be done – at least while the person is sucking on the lollipop. Playing music that the person enjoys is another distracter to bathing.

- **Create a safe and pleasing atmosphere.** Provide non-slip adhesives on the floor surface and grab bars in the bathtub to prevent falls and provide security. Provide a pleasant, clean aroma and indirect lighting.
- **Use a shower chair with a 7-foot long shower hose** so it is possible to rinse all parts of the person – be careful not to get water in the person's eyes.
- **Make the Bathroom a Safer and Friendlier Place for those with Alzheimer's** – these suggestions are important for managing urinating and defecating but also bathing and brushing teeth as well.

1. Cover or remove wall to wall mirrors – seeing the reflections in the mirror confuses the person with AD who might have trouble determining whether there are strangers in the room – this may precipitate a catastrophic reaction where the person with AD and/or the caregiver gets hurt.   Mirrors that are on a medicine cabinet do not generate the same response.
2. Change knobs, which are associated with burns, to handles on sinks and tubs.
3. Remove glass sliding doors – they are an accident waiting to happen. Replace with a rod and use a sturdy cotton duct curtain with metal grommets that can't be torn through.

- **Respect the person's dignity.** Allow the person to hold a towel in front of the body while being bathed - Both in and out of the shower if desired. This may ease anxiety.
- **Don't worry about the frequency of bathing.** It may not be necessary to bathe every day. Sponge baths can be effective between showers and baths.
- **Be gentle.** The person's skin may be very sensitive, so avoid scrubbing and pat skin dry instead of rubbing.
- **Be flexible.** The person may experience the most difficulty when caregiver is attempting to shower his/her head or shampoo his/her hair. If this is the case, avoid spraying water on his/her head; use a washcloth to soap and rinse hair, reducing the amount of water on the person's face.

SECTION 4

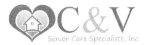

DRESSING WITHOUT A BATTLE

The person with dementia may present problems with dressing him/herself. The person may choose to wear the same outfit every day, may choose to wear clothing that is not clean, may attempt to dress at inappropriate times during the day or night, or in the later stages may have difficulty figuring out how to put on a piece of clothing. These behaviors occur because the person no longer clearly understands the cultural norms for dressing or no longer has the attention to detail to recognize that clothing is soiled, or has become confused about the daily schedule or routine, or has lost the ability to sequence putting on different garments.

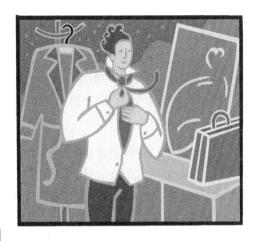

Try the Following:

- **Simplify selection** by reducing the number of available garments to 2 or 3 and group into ready-to-wear combinations.
- **Choose comfortable and simple clothing.** Substitute Velcro for buttons or zippers when possible, or assist with fasteners. Make sure shoes are comfortable and support the foot and ankle.
- **Minimize distractions.** Turn off the TV or music. Provide adequate lighting.
- **Be flexible.** If the individual wants to wear the same outfit repeatedly, try getting a duplicate of the outfit or have similar options available.
- **Follow a strict routine.** Develop a schedule that allows the person to dress for the day and undress for the evening at specific fixed times.
- **Be individual.** Allow 2-3 times the usual time to dress.
- **Organize the process.** Lay out clothing in the order it needs to be put on, or hand the person each piece while giving short, simple instructions.

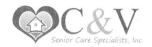

TIPS FOR BRUSHING TEETH

Sometimes it is helpful to say, "Mom, WE need to brush OUR teeth" instead of you need to brush your teeth. Or, "Mom, why don't WE brush OUR teeth together?" or "Mom, I want to be sure that OUR teeth stay nice and healthy, why don't WE brush our teeth".

It is also helpful to use the kitchen sink. Get out two toothbrushes and two tubes of toothpaste Use the same brand of toothpaste the person has always used, if you can. <u>Organize before you suggest that the person needs to brush his/her teeth.</u> Apply toothpaste to the brush for him/her. Provide a thick-handled, easy-to-grip toothbrush.

Get the person with Alzheimer's strategically set, standing right in front of her/his toothbrush and toothpaste which is sitting strategically right next to the sink.

Turn on the water. The caregiver needs to pick up her/his brush, and start brushing. This action is a demonstration of what to do.

The caregiver doesn't encourage or cajole the person to brush – the caregiver just continues to: Brush. Spit. Brush.

Finally, it is good for the caregiver to make a short comment such as "This feels good. I don't want to end up in the dentist's chair, this is why I am brushing."

The caregiver needs to continue brushing, spitting, and smiling in between without saying a word.

Then the caregiver puts down his/her brush and picks up the brush of the person with Alzheimer's. Next the caregiver puts some toothpaste on the brush and hands the brush over without saying a word but while smiling. . Remember, many Alzheimer's individuals can only do one thing at a time. They can't multi-task - this means they can't talk and brush their teeth at the same time.

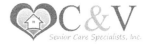

If the person with Alzheimer's doesn't brush, or if they say something negative, move the brush a little bit so they can see it, and don't say a word. Smile. Relax. Smile.

Finally, it's up to the caregiver to walk away.

The more you talk, cajole, or make negative comments the less chance you have of getting the person with Alzheimer's to brush – the fewer words used the better. This technique may work immediately or it might take several months – you must be patient and positive.

DeMarco. B. 2011. *http://www.alzheimersreadingroom.com/2011/05/how-to-get-alzheimers-individual-to brush.html*, Accessed July 15, 2012.

SHAMPOOING HAIR

- If caregiver is washing the person's hair, a hand-held shower may work best.

- Think about using a shampoo which will not cause stinging if it gets into the person's eyes or using a hair wash shield to prevent water running onto the person's face. Another option is a 'no rinse' shampoo that can clean the hair without using water.

- If the person prefers to have her/his hair washed by a hairdresser, either arrange trips to the salon, or find a hairdresser who will come to the house. This may be a time when the caregiver can have her/his hair cut too.

- There are a number of products to make shampooing of hair easier. Carepathways.com sells an EZ-Shampoo Deluxe Basin; an EZ Shampoo Shower, and a Hair Washing Tray

http://www.activeforever.com/s-16-bathing-aids-hygiene.aspx
Active Forever has great bathing devices that can be used.

http://shop.alzstore.com/bathing-c16.aspx
The Alzheimer's store has bathing and wandering prevention devices.

http://www.caregiverproducts.com/site/270651/page/911684
Caregiver Products.com has several bathing and hair washing aides.

http://www.amazon.com/s/?ie=UTF8&keywords=bath+hat&tag=mh0b-20&index=baby&hvadid=56811291&ref=pd_sl_4a8fxk5ym4_b
*Amazon has numerous "bath hats" for children that prevent water from getting in a child's eyes. These could be used for adults (BESTEK drain stopper hat shampoo cap bath hat shower cap baby shower accessories baby hair shampoo and body wash cap sun hat BTSC101, Rinse Splashguard , Dry Eyes Shampoo Visor).

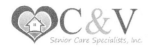

PROMOTING ADEQUATE SLEEP

It is very common for the person with Alzheimer's to get her/his "days and nights mixed up". Although it is not possible for the caregiver to totally control this there are a number of strategies to promote adequate sleep. These include:

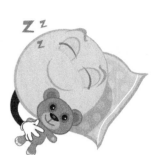

- Providing physical exercise during the daytime
- Establishing a night time routine —e.g brushing teeth, washing face, taking a warm bath or shower, praying, reading or using relaxation techniques.
- Providing a light nutritious snack prior to bed
- Providing a glass of warm milk before bed
- Avoiding caffeine and nicotine especially in the evening hours
- Engaging in a relaxing activity prior to bedtime
- Remaining on a schedule or routine during the day facilitates sleep at night.
- Administering sleep medications as prescribed

If the individual continues to get up during the night even though you have implemented all the above suggestions, then you need to make sure that the person is safe when up and roaming about.

- Consider purchasing an infrared eye alarm that beeps when the individual crosses the threshold of the bedroom.
- Purchase a baby monitor and place one in the person's room and one in the bedroom of the caregiver so that the individual falling or calling for help will be heard.
- Make sure the individual cannot get out of the house. Locks need to be placed out of the line of vision – either very high or very low. In addition, double bolt door locks should be used to the outside – keep the key easily accessible in case of an emergency.
- Place the person with Alzheimer's in a bedroom with the mattress on the floor to prevent falls getting out of bed.
- Make sure there is a night light in the individual's room.
- Keep lights on in hallways.
- Don't lock the person in his/her room.
- Where there are stairs a barrier such as a door needs to be placed at the top of stairs. At the bottom of the stairs a baby gate works well – Those with Alzheimer's usually can't open the gate or step over the gate.

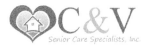

- Make sure the person can not turn on the stove.
- Be prepared in case wandering does occur. Have a current picture of the person with Alzheimer's along with accurate information regarding height, weight, color of hair and other identifiers that will increase the chances that the individual will be found quickly. Make sure that neighbors aware that this person is memory impaired and that if this individual is seen wandering outside of the home to please invite him/her in for a drink of water and to call the family.
- Make sure the person with AD can not access poisons or matches or other substances that may pose a risk. For additional suggestions, see the teaching tools, "Ways to ensure fire and burn safety" and "Ways to store dangerous substances".

EXERCISE IS NOT A DIRTY WORD

Until the very advanced stages of AD, most people with the disease have the physical ability, energy, and desire to get some form of exercise. What they often need is assistance in identifying safe forms of exercise, and then initiating and completing the exercise consistently.

Exercise offers many benefits to older people, such as better sleep, improved strength and balance, less constipation, and improved mood and individuals with AD are no exception. For instance, for the AD individual who is losing many abilities, physical fitness is one area where he or she can actually show improvement. Studies also show that regular exercise reduces the occurrence of undesirable behaviors such as wandering, pulling at clothing, and regression. Participation in exercise can actually make caregiving easier in the long run.

A physical therapist can design a balanced exercise program that is suitable and safe for the individual, but here are some general tips for successful exercise:

- A major key in keeping an exercise program going is having a "coach" or "buddy". This may be the spouse, a friend, or neighbor, a hired caregiver or family member who walks or exercises with the individual.

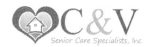

- Exercise needs to be a routine, whether it is daily or 3 times a week. It helps to follow a routine walking path or a regimen of exercises. Keep the same sequence every time and try to do it at the same time of the day.
- Walking is the easiest and the most readily available form of exercise and it can be combined with walking the dog, getting the mail, or other purposeful activities. Something familiar to the individual, such as dancing, stationary bike or tossing a ball is good.
- Set very realistic, short term goals, such as increasing time on the stationary bike by one minute/per week.
- Exercise along with your loved one. It's good for you, too!
- Use simple instructions and touch or pointing to guide the individual. "Turn this way" instead of "turn to your left."
- Try sitting or "chair" exercises if balance is a concern.
- Try to include some gentle stretching, balance activities, strengthening exercises and aerobic exercise. If the individual has been inactive, the goal is to establish a regular exercise program. If the individual is already active, the goal is to continue or increase activity to 30 minutes or more of moderate intensity.

ENJOYING YOUR LOVED ONE
BECOMING AN ALZHEIMER'S WHISPERER®
THROUGH ACTIVITIES

Activities are the things that we do, who we are and what we're about. These activities include getting dressed, doing chores, and even paying bills. For the person with Alzheimer's, they can mean the difference between thinking loved and needed and unloved and unnecessary.

In planning activities for your loved one it is essential to remember:

1) You can change your response to her/his behavior; he/she cannot change behavior for you.
2) You can enter the person with AD's reality; she/he cannot be pulled into yours.
3) "One size does not fit all" when comes to what will or will not work for each individual.
4) No technique is 100% fail-proof; must be flexible.

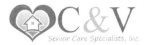

5) It is important to allow them person with AD a sense of participating in the normal activities of life.
6) Success means adapting the task to the individual's ability at whatever level that ability may be.
7) The process is more important than the result; celebrate the process not the result.

When planning activities and daily tasks to help the person with Alzheimer's organize the day, think about:

- What skills and abilities does the person have?
- What does the person enjoy doing?
- Does the person begin activities without direction?
- Does the person have physical problems?

Your approach

- Make the activities part of the daily routine.
- Focus on enjoyment, not achievement.
- Determine what time of date is best for the activity.

Offer support and supervision.

- Be flexible with individual, and stress involvement.
- Help the person remain as independent as possible.
- Simplify instructions.
- Establish a familiar routine.

The environment
I.e. make activities safe.

- Change your surroundings to encourage activities.
- Minimize distractions that can frighten or confuse the person.
- Structuring the day –**BUILD IN LOTS OF OPPORTUNITIES FOR SNACKS AND DRINKS**

When structuring the day, consider the following activities:

Morning activities

- Wash up, brush teeth, and get dressed.
- Prepare and eat breakfast.

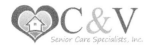

- Discuss the newspaper or reminisce about old photos.

Afternoon activities

- Prepare and eat lunch, read mail, and clear and wash dishes.
- Listen to music or do a crossword puzzle.
- Take a walk.

Evening activities

- Prepare and eat dinner.
- Play cards or watch a movie
- Read a book or magazine

Activities that enhance the quality of life must be dignified, safe, adaptable, repetitious, and interesting to the individual.

In early Alzheimer's disease, the individual can probably still do his or her own personal care. A person who has always loved working in his yard may enjoy raking leaves. Someone who loves cooking may enjoy working in her kitchen. If she can no longer operate the stove safely, the caregiver could suggest preparing foods that do not require cooking such as cold sandwiches, or salads.

In middle Alzheimer's there are a few techniques that caregivers will find useful. One technique is called "cueing." Because the disease interferes the individual's ability to think, reason, and remember, simple activities such as taking off shirt can be too confusing. "Cueing" involves breaking each task down into its various and verbalizing them to your loved one. For instance, you would say, "Unbutton your shirt. When that step is completed, you would say, "Slip it off this shoulder." Then, you would continue, "Now slide your arm out." Each step of the process would follow until the task is completed. Rather than have you take his shirt off, your loved one has removed it himself.

Another technique useful in the middle stage is called "mirroring." This is a technique where caregivers model the activity they want their loved one to do. Caregivers might pretend to brush their hair or raise an imaginary glass to their lips. Seeing the action often causes individuals with Alzheimer's to imitate what their caregivers pretend to do.

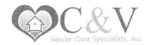

In late-stage Alzheimer's disease some different techniques are needed. These include "hand over hand," "chaining," and "end chaining." In "hand over hand," caregivers place their hands over the hands of the person with Alzheimer's to guide them in the activity. This can be done for washing the body and brushing teeth. "Chaining" is when caregivers begin an activity with the "hand over" technique, but after their loved one has performed the activity for a short time, the guiding hands are removed. The individual may continue the activity alone. In "end chaining," the caregiver begins the activity and then stops abruptly at an uncomfortable stage, causing individual to complete the activity in order to restore comfort. For example, the caregiver might begin to brush the individual's teeth, then remove his or her hand from the mouth with the toothbrush left hanging out of the mouth, the individual will generally reach up to grasp it and, oftentimes, then begin brushing independently.

In the very last stage of the disease, "sensory bridging" might help to maintain the individual's sense of participating in the activities of his or her life. Examples of "sensory bridging" would be placing a wash cloth and/or lotion bottle in the loved one's hands while being bathed or a napkin or spoon while being fed. Any of these techniques can be tried at home by caregivers who want to enhance the quality of life for their family member.

Outside Activities for the Person with Dementia

Outside activities can be relaxing, fulfilling, and give your loved one a sense of self-worth. The more active they are during the days the more peaceful the evenings and nights can be. Remember to enjoy your time together, relax and have fun!

The following are ideas for outside activities as well as the benefits that these activities provide.

- Help put plants or bulbs in small pots, or pull old plants and weeds from the garden. This will provide a sense of accomplishment.
- Look at flowers and plants together.
- Reminisce about playing barefoot in the dirt as a child, or what he/she remembers about what it was like when she/he were children playing outside. Most people with Alzheimer's disease are able to reminisce and enjoy doing so.

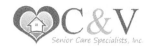

- Plant a small garden. This activity can be enjoyed all spring and summer. You and your loved one can check your garden daily for new sprouts or ripe vegetables. This activity can also lead to other activities such as picking and preparing what they have grown in their garden.
- Animal watching. Put a birdbath and feeders out in the yard. Your loved one can keep feeders full and water in the bath.
- Picnic Lunch. Have a special lunch or snack outside. Sip on fresh lemonade or an ice cream cone. Take some old family photos and listen to oldies. This can be relaxing for both of you, as well as bring back fond memories.
- Reading. Sit outside under the shade and read poetry or books of short memoirs. Short stories or poems do not have to be remembered to enjoy them.
- Pick up leaves, rocks, flowers or grass. Talk about the differences in the way they feel or smell. This is wonderful sensory stimulation. It can also lead to reminiscing.
- Other outdoor activities. Horseshoes, water plants and flowers, pick weeds; sweep the porch, plant window boxes and more!

Use of Music

Often, memories -of the person with Alzheimer's disease can be stimulated through music. Songs from different stages of life can bring back old memories and help the person think more alive in the present. Love songs are very popular because many people can relate to those thoughts. Classics are available at music stores or the local library. Try listening to these songs with your loved one:

> *Let Me Call You. Sweetheart*
> *When I Grow Too Old To Dream*
> *Somewhere My Love*
> *Give Me A Little Kiss (Will You?)*
> *Be My Love*
> *Are You Lonesome Tonight*
> *I Love You Truly*
> *Heart Of My Heart*
> *Release Me*
> *Goodnight Sweetheart*

- Sing-Alongs are also good activities. With the choice of proper songs, orientation to place and time can be promoted. Choose songs to sing

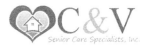

together such as "Deep in the Heart of Texas", "if You Knew Susie", or "White Christmas." Also consider using rhythm when having a sing-along. Simple instruments can be made from coffee cans or shaking beans.

- Use live music, tapes, or CDs; radio programs, interrupted by too many commercials, can cause confusion.
- Use music to create the mood you want.
- Link music with other reminiscence activities; use questions or photographs to help stir memories.
- Encourage movement (clapping, dancing) to add to the enjoyment.
- Avoid sensory overload; eliminate competing noises by shutting windows and doors and by turning off the television.

Art as an Activity

In using Art as an activity, the caregiver must "assume" the individual has many things he/she would like to say and that there is some meaning in what people say or do, no matter how garbled verbal expression might be. It also assumes she/he can do more than they have been given credit for to date, and it gently challenges him/her as well.

There is no right or wrong in art and there should not be a "color within the lines attitude." By following simple guidelines, the person with Alzheimer's will create art work that leads to happy attitudes.

Start each session like a happy visit; Focus on creativity, not technique; Perceive their pictures as stories (not the daffodil they drew, but the daffodil they picked from their mother's garden); remain open to new images; Encourage sociability; Be flexible; Don't push; Use humor and appreciate their humor; and Listen for their poetry.

Create a relaxed, non-judgmental environment for engaging in artwork by:
- Being prepared ahead of time so as not to hurry the artist;
- Use conversation and make explanations simple;
- Expect the person with AD to forget;
- Maintain a relaxed tempo as the activity progresses;
- Make instructions short, maintaining a non-judgemental attitude

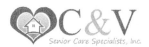

- Be supportive; Provide encouragement, discuss what the person is creating, and try to initiate a bit of creative storytelling or reminiscence.

- Try to think and work in the world of the person with AD; and be prepared and organized but do not expect your loved one to be flexible.

- Help the person begin the activity. If the person is painting, you may need to start the brush movement. Most other projects should only require basic instruction and assistance.

- Use safe materials. Avoid toxic substances and sharp tools. Allow plenty of time to complete the art project.

- The person doesn't have to finish the project in one sitting.

  And remember: The artwork is complete when the person says it is.

Massage and Touch

Often, as the person with Alzheimer's disease becomes more withdrawn and less verbal in communication, non-verbal communication becomes very important. We have known that babies who do not have their physical needs met will still die unless they are also emotionally -nurtured through touch. That need continues throughout life. Ashley Montague wrote, "The use of touch and physical closeness may be the most important way to communicate to acutely ill persons that they are important as human beings."'

Physical and emotional pain can often be eased with massage. Physical pain is often increased when muscles are tense; massage can relax those muscles. The very act of touching through massage alleviates some feelings of isolation and abandonment many Alzheimer's individuals experience. Because massage is very relaxing, in some instances, it can eliminate sleeplessness and the need for sleep medication.

Aroma

Many memories are made from associations with smell. The use of aroma can increase stimulation, enhance memory association, stimulate conversation promote mood stabilization. It uses essential oils drawn from seeds, berries, barks, petals, and resins in a variety of applications to influence individual's moods. These applications include massage dispersing the oils through a diffuser, a lamp ring, a spray bottle or a cotton boutonniere.

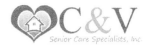

There are simple guidelines to follow when using aroma:
1) Never apply essential oils on the skin.
2) Always dilute in lotion, oil, water or in the air.
3) Observe for sensitivities and allergic reactions, such as nausea, lightheadedness and redness of skin -- discontinue of that particular oil.
4) Do not use oils for long extended time frames.

To influence moods, the following essential oils can be used by the caregiver:

- Invigorating: Peppermint, rosemary, lemon
- Relaxing: Chamomile, marjoram, ylang-ylang
- Sedating: Lavender, juniper, sandalwood
- Mentally clarifying: Clary sage, fennel, basil
- Depression - lifting: Grapefruit, rose
- Immunity - strengthening: Bergamot, tea tree, cajuput
- Anxiety - lifting: Orange, jasmine, frankincense

What else can you do?

- Make a memory book, a personal scrapbook. Look at it and read it out loud a lot!
- Fold laundry. (This can happen over and over again if it's a hit.)
- Make cookies. (This also can happen over and over again!)
- Collect catalogues and newspaper shopping ads and go "wish book" shopping.
- Compare prices then and now. Talk about rationing.
- Collect and sort nuts and washers and bolts of different sizes.
- Plant and tend a windowsill herb garden.
- Test small batteries with a portable battery tester.
- Rearrange drawers.
- Rearrange them tomorrow, too!
- Read the personal ads in the paper. Make up your own!
- Sweep the porch and the walk.
- Hard boil aging eggs and make deviled eggs or egg salad.
- Get a handbook for simple dice games and play. Yahtzee too!
- Go to fabric stores or hardware stores and browse the trims and gadgets.

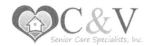

- Play alphabet games with household container labels. Look for all 26 letters on a label.
- Collect postcards and stamps, old and new. Send postcards to loved ones. Ask your librarian to help you find poems and primers that date back to- school days.
- Look out the window or sit on the porch. Count the colors or makes of cars that go by.
- Scrub the sinks in the house. Wash the windows, too!
- Watch a musical on video every week. Watch in 30 minute segments if necessary.
- Make apple pie or cobbler from scratch. See who can peel the longest unbroken peel!
- Make candy cane decorations from pipe cleaners and red & white beads.
- Soak feet and give a foot massage. Paint toenails if desired!
- Have a happy hour with music and salsa and chips and margarita mix, without alcohol.
- Put up maps of the state, country and world. Mark important places.
- Put up a family timeline on the walls of a room - births, deaths, moves, marriages, etc.
- Brush each other's hair. Lotion each other's hands. Rub each other's shoulders.
- Polish and shine shoes.
- Make birthday card collages for loved ones from old magazines.
- Put on some favorite, irresistible music and MOVE! (You don't have to call it dancing!)
- Ask for advice about a problem. Really <u>listen.</u>
- Read and recite favorite poems.
- Sing favorite hymns and carols
- Play a name game - list as many girls and boys names for each alphabet letter as you can
- Blow up an inflatable punch ball and use it as indoor balloon volleyball.
- Wipe countertops and cupboards and doors and light switches and trim.
- Take a walk and read the mailboxes, road signs and business signs out loud.
- Watch a talk show (or a shock - talk show) together. Express your opinions!

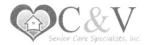

SECTION 5

SAFETY CONCERNS

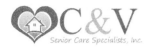

WANDERING: WHY IT OCCURS
AND HOW TO DEAL WITH IT

An individual with Alzheimer's is likely to wander at some point during the disease. This is an incredibly stressful behavior for loved ones to deal with because of the safety implications associated with wandering. Sometimes people wander because they have a need to get somewhere specific- a job they once held, an appointment or to go "home". Sometimes the wandering is aimless and the goal is just to "get out" without a specific destination in mind.

The first approach is to try to identify why your loved one is wandering. There may be a number of causes, including:

- Medication Side effects
- Stress
- Confusion related to time
- Restlessness
- Agitation
- Inability to recognize familiar people, places and objects
- Fear arising from the misinterpretation of sights and sounds
- Desire to fulfill former obligations, such as going to work or looking after a child

Tips for reducing wandering behavior:

- Encourage movement and exercise to reduce anxiety, agitation, and restlessness
- Involve your loved one in productive daily activities such as folding laundry or preparing dinner
- Remind your loved one he is in the right place
- Reassure him if he thinks lost, abandoned, or disoriented.

Tips for protecting your loved one from wandering:

- Enroll the person in the Alzheimer's Association's Safe Return Program
- Check with your local police and fire departments to see if they are giving away GPS bracelets that your loved one would wear and could be tracked if he/she wandered.
- Use black or brown rugs taped down with electrical tape in front of all exterior doors and also the door that might lead to a basement – the person

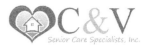

with Alzheimer's frequently misperceives the dark rug as a hole and will not step over it.

- Move the deadbolt locks to the top of the doors – the person with Alzheimer's has a narrow range of vision
- Have an up to date picture of your loved one with description of height, weight and distinguishing features.
- Camouflaging door knobs by covering them with material that is the same color as the walls
- Placing movable screens or curtains in front of doors also makes them "disappear" to the person with AD.
- Planning activities around the times when the person with AD is most restless and inclined to wander is another important strategy.
- If the individual is a night wanderer it is essential that the stove is disabled, that medications, cleaning supplies and other potentially toxic substances are safely secured, and that there is adequate lighting so the person with AD is less likely to fall and be injured.

Additional interventions to limit night wandering include restricting fluids two hours prior to bedtime and ensuring that the individual with AD has gone to the bathroom before going to bed. Limiting daytime naps also helps to limit nighttime wandering.

- Inform your neighbors of the person's condition and keep a list of their names and telephone numbers
- Keep your home safe and secure by installing deadbolt locks on exterior doors and limiting access to potentially dangerous areas
- Be aware that the person may not only wander by foot but also by other modes of transportation.
- **Be aware that the individual who is wandering usually takes off toward his/her dominant side.**

Tips for preparing for emergencies

- Keep list of emergency phone numbers and addresses of the local police and fire departments, hospitals, and poison control as well as Safe Return help lines.
- Check fire extinguishers and smoke alarms, and conduct fire drills regularly.

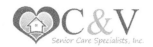

THE SAFE RETURN PROGRAM

Safe Return is a national, government funded program of the Alzheimer's Association that assists in the identification and safe return of individuals with Alzheimer's Disease and related dementias who wander off, sometimes far from home, and become lost.

The Alzheimer's Association's Safe Return Program is the only nationwide program of its kind. It began in 1993. Since then nearly 100,000 individuals have registered in Safe Return nationwide. The program has facilitated the return of more than 7,500 individuals to their families and caregivers with an over 99% success in returning those registered in the program.

How Does Safe Return Work?

The Safe Return Program helps unite families by working through Alzheimer's Association chapters across the country and trained community members like law enforcement officials, emergency medical technicians, and transit operators. The program includes:

- Identification products including wallet cards, jewelry, clothing labels, lapel pin, and bag tags
- A national photo/information database
- A 24-hour toll-free crisis line
- Alzheimer's Association local chapter support
- Wandering behavior education and training for caregivers and families

If the registrant wanders and is found, the person who finds him/her can call the Safe Return toll free number located on the wanderer's identification wallet card, jewelry, or clothing labels. The Safe Return telephone operator immediately alerts the family members or caregiver listed in the database, so they can be reunited with their loved one.

If a person is reported missing by a family member or caregiver, Safe Return can fax law enforcement agencies the missing person's information and photograph. Local Alzheimer's Association Chapters provide family support and assistance while police conduct the search and rescue. To register, a person with dementia or their caregiver fills out a simple form, supplies a photograph, and chooses the type of identification product that the registrant will wear and/or carry.

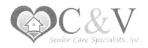

For:

$55 + $7 shipping and handling, you receive an enrollment package including:

Member's ID jewelry with personalized information and MedicAlert + Safe Return's 24-hour emergency toll-free number

Personalized emergency wallet card

24-hour emergency response service

Personal health record (PHR)

Six Steps to a Safe Return magnet

(Optional) Add $35 for caregiver ID jewelry and membership

Membership includes everything listed above.

The caregiver wears this worldwide-recognized ID jewelry to alert others that he or she provides care for a MedicAlert + Safe Return member, in case of an emergency

$35 annual renewal fee
An annual fee of $35 will be due after the first year for each membership.

Read more: *http://www.alz.org/care/dementia-medic-alert-safe-return.asp#ixzz3AmTwUZZp*

When registering on-line or by phone, you will be asked to provide the following information:
- Registrant's name and contact information
- Registrant's identifying characteristics (Social Security #, height, weight, eye color, distinguishing marks and characteristics, etc.)
- Registrant's EXACT wrist measurement in inches (required when ordering a bracelet).
- Up to three contact names, addresses, and phone numbers
- Local law enforcement information (address, phone, and fax numbers)
- Credit Card number and expiration date

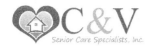

To register by phone using a credit care, call 888-572-8566
Monday through Friday 8 a.m. to 8 p.m. Central Time.

To register on line go to *www.alz.org*

To register by mail, complete the registration form and return to:

Safe Return

P.O. Box 9307

St. Louis, Missouri 63117-0307

It is also important to check with Police and Fire Departments in your area – an increasing number of these across the nation are providing GPS bracelets.

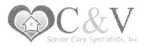

THE DEAR NEIGHBOR LETTER

Date

Dear Neighbors:

You may not know that my_____

whose name is_____,

and lives at_____ is memory impaired.

As a result, _____sometimes loses track of

Where _____ lives. _____may wander off and become lost or

confused.

You may see _____ in your yard or walking by your

house. _____poses no danger to you, but may say things you

cannot make sense of or behave erratically. I would appreciate it if you

could approach _____gently and

quietly.

If you don't ask _____too many questions, but suggest

that _____come inside for a drink of water, or let

you bring _____one, you may be able to detain

_____while you call me at _____.

I will come and get _____immediately. This is a challenging

problem, and it's not possible for me to police _____'s

activities all the time. I can't tell you how much I appreciate your help if the

need arises.

Sincerely,

_____

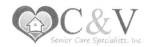

WAYS TO ENSURE FIRE AND BURN SAFETY

Fire and burn safety are critically important and take on two dimensions with the Alzheimer's individual. The first dimension is minimizing the risks that the individual will start a fire. This is done by locking away matches, lighters and lighter fluid.

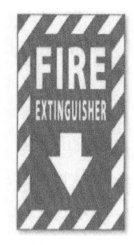

However the most important intervention is to disable the stove when there is no one around who can provide supervision. The individual can still have access to food but should not be given access to a working stove. Stoves pose more of a fire risk for individuals than anything else. Perhaps the lifelong habit of cooking makes them turn to use the stove. Remember the stove must be disabled!

The second dimension deals with protecting the individual from accidental burns and making sure the individual is safe in case there is a house fire. The following are "must do" interventions:

- Turn down the temperature on the water heater so that the individual is not accidentally burned while in the tub/shower or using the faucet.
- Have a working fire alarm in the house- make sure it is tested and battery replaced as needed.
- The home should be equipped with fire extinguishers

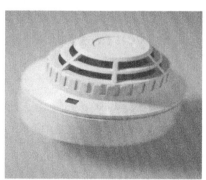

- Contact the local fire department – they frequently supply stickers indicating "child" or "handicapped person" – these stickers should be placed in the corner of the individual's bedroom window. This alerts first responders to an emergency that there is a person in that room who can not get out independently.
- If person lives in an apartment building or a group home the manager must have a plan for assisting residents who suffer from memory impairment to a place of safety.

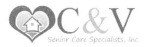

WAYS TO STORE DANGEROUS SUBSTANCES

Take a walk through the home – look through closets, cupboards, underneath sinks, and other places where substances might be stored. Gather them up and place them in an area that can be locked up. Any substance including cleaning supplies that could harm the individual if ingested must be locked up. This would include all medications.

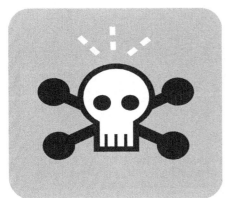

Sometimes cleaning supplies look like drinks and are very inviting to the person who no longer has the ability to distinguish between Windex and Gator Aid. Medications can be mistaken for candy- as you walk through your house ask yourself: "What would I put away in a safe place if I had a toddler in the house?" Those are exactly the products that need to be placed in a safe place if you are caring for someone with Alzheimer's disease

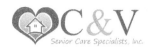

WAYS TO PREVENT DRIVING

Driving is a complex activity that demands quick reactions, alert senses, and split-second decision making. For a person with Alzheimer's, driving inevitably becomes difficult.

A diagnosis of Alzheimer's disease does not mean the person has lost all ability to drive. Caregivers should evaluate the person regularly to determine if it is safe for him or her to drive.

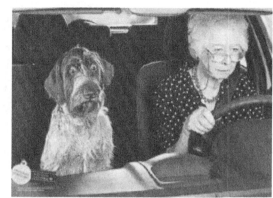

Warning signs of unsafe driving
- Forgetting how to locate familiar places
- Failing to observe traffic signals
- Making slow or poor decisions
- Driving at an inappropriate speed
- Becoming angry and confused while driving

For many, restricting driving privileges signifies a loss of independence and mobility, often forcing people with the disease to rely on friends, family, and community services for transportation. This sense of dependence may prevent people with dementia from giving up the car keys.

Tips on preventing a person with Alzheimer's from driving

- Ask a doctor to write a "do not drive" prescription
- Ask doctor to recommend a driving safety test offered by most MVA's
- Have the person tested by the Department of Motor Vehicles
- Control access to the car keys
- Disable the car by removing the distributor cap or battery
- Park the car on another block or in a neighbor's driveway
- Arrange for other transportation
- Substitute the person's driver's license with a photo identification card (in addition to making the car inaccessible)

Be sensitive and supportive during this non-driving transition, when the person may become angry and depressed.

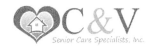

SECTION 6

CHALLENGING BEHAVIORS

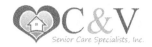

DEALING WITH CHALLENGING BEHAVIORS

Always start with the 4 "R"s when responding to a person with Alzheimer's disease:

1. Reassess
2. Rechannel
3. Reassure
4. Reconsider

REASSESS: When confronted with challenging behaviors, ask the following questions:

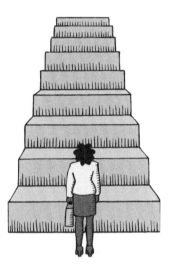

1. Is there a reason for this behavior? Physical or Pain
2. Is the individual frustrated because of his/her inability to do something?
3. Is he/she uncomfortable about a situation?
4. Is there too much noise?
5. Is there too much activity going?
6. Or, is there TO LITTLE stimulation?

RECHANNEL: If the person is doing something annoying then try to redirect them by:
1. Give the person something to do.
2. Fold clothes.
3. Straighten magazines.
4. Push in chairs; wipe off tables, And if it is an annoying behavior, like throwing out the newspaper – then hide today's paper and leave out yesterday's paper – BE CREATIVE!

REASSURE: The Alzheimer's individual lives in a world he/she no longer understand; where people do things to him/her that he/she does not understand; he/she may not recognize many people- even the people that she/he lives with; the environment is too noisy or too busy or too hurried. People with AD need lots of reassurance. Talk to them with soothing words, or a tender touch- even a pat on the back or a hug can make them feel so much better. You are offering comfort and assurance that everything is okay. ***Remember his/her memory might be gone but he/she still has feelings but may lack the ability to express these feelings.***
RECONSIDER: Try seeing the world from the individual's perspective.

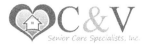

So much of what they are expected to do is a challenge – nothing seems normal. Most of the people they see are strangers; the world is incomprehensible to them. Every one speaks a language that they don't understand. Can you imagine how difficult this must be?

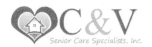

REPETITIVE BEHAVIORS

The individual asks the same question over and over again, or they do the same thing over and over again. It's enough to make you crazy! First of all make sure he/she is not in pain or hungry. If there is no pain and the person is not hungry you **DISTRACT!**

- Take the individual for a walk
- Give the individual a snack
- Play music – sing a song
- Make up a song describing the situation – use a tune with which the individual is familiar
- Give the individual something physical to do
  - Rolling coins
  - Folding towels
  - Sweeping
- Or, try your best to ignore it.

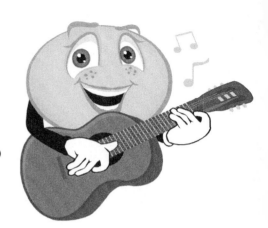

HALLUCINATIONS

Hallucinations are another common problem that develops in Alzheimer's. The individual thinks, sees, hears, smells, or tastes something that isn't there. You deal with this in a number of ways. If the hallucination doesn't cause problems for the individual, for you, for other family members, you might want to ignore it. However if the individual is continuously hallucinating, consult the physician to make sure there is not any underlying physical cause. Also, have the individual's eyesight and hearing checked and make sure the individual wears his or her glasses or hearing aid on a regular basis.

Offer reassurance. Hallucinations may be frightening to the individual. Never argue with the individual. It is not helpful to tell the individual that something is not real. So if the content of the hallucination is pleasant, e.g. "My mother is coming for dinner." Then say, "Really? I know you'll have a wonderful time." If the hallucination is frightening then you have to address it in a way that recognizes and allays the individual's fear. For example, the individual says, "There is a mean dog in my room." Instead of saying, "No there's not" say instead, "Really! Well I can see why you're afraid. But don't worry I won't let it hurt you."

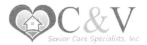

It is not uncommon for an individual to get frightened by looking in a mirror and seeing his/her own reflection. However, the individual is afraid because he doesn't recognize the face staring back at him. Reassure and cover the mirrors.

Other approaches to hallucinations include: suggest that the individual walk or sit in another room. Frightening hallucinations often subside in well-lit areas where other people are present.

Try to turn the individual's attention to music, conversation or activities that you enjoy together.

SUNDOWNING

Sundowning is a symptom that results in increased confusion, anxiety, agitation and disorientation. It sometimes begins in the late afternoon and can extend into the evening. No one really knows why it happens but factors such as fatigue, reduced lighting and increased shadows, and other factors may contribute to Sundowning. What do we do to reduce the evening agitation?
1. Plan more active days – take a walk or engage in other physical activity
2. Restrict caffeine consumption to the morning hours.
3. Reduce the number of things going on in the environment
4. Keep distractions to a minimum
5. Limit activities during the late afternoon and early evening to those that are simple and relaxing
6. If the individual begins to pace, keep an eye on him– don't try to stop the individual- it may precipitate a catastrophic outburst.

SCREAMING AND CATASTROPHIC OUTBURSTS
Most of the time a catastrophic outburst is expressed through crying. However, sometimes the crying is accompanied by other behaviors including violence.

If the individual becomes verbally abusive:
1. Try to ignore it.
2. Look for the reason it is happening – too much noise? Too much activity?
3. Try distraction – change the subject, offer a treat.
4. Maintain a calm and soothing approach.
5. Don't argue

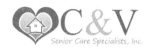

For a physical outburst:
1. If you feel threatened walk away.
2. Don't try to remove the person from the area without assistance – make sure you protect yourself and any other person who might be in harm's way
3. Remove any objects that could be used as a weapon- book, wheelchair or walker
4. Give the individual plenty of space when you approach
5. Move towards the individual very slowly and very cautiously
6. Make eye contact with the individual
7. And if you don't know that it's safe, stay back and hold out your hand in a non-threatening manner. Time for the 5th "R".... if you think you are in danger RETREAT

AGITATION AND AGGRESSION

Agitated Behaviors: In the early stages of Alzheimer's disease people may experience:
1. Personality changes such as irritability,
2. Anxiety, or
3. Depression.

As the disease progresses, other symptoms may occur, including:
1. Sleep disturbances,
2. Delusions (firmly held beliefs in things that are not real),
3. Hallucinations (see above),
4. Pacing,
5. Constant movement or restlessness,
6. Checking or rechecking door locks or appliances, tearing tissues,
7. General emotional outbursts, and
8. Cursing or threatening language.

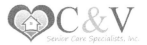

Causes of Agitation

1. Pain-Assess
2. Medical conditions and drug interactions that may worsen person's thinking ability
3. Changes in individual's situation such as moving to new residence or nursing home
4. Changes in caregiver arrangements,
5. Environmental changes
6. Misperceived threats
7. Fear and fatigue from trying to make sense out of a confusing world

Treating Agitation

1. Medical evaluation- especially when agitation comes on suddenly
2. If a medical problem underlying agitation – appropriate treatment may deal with agitation
3. Behavioral treatments identify the behavior, try to understand the cause, and adapt the caregiving environment to improve the situation.
4. Good record keeping helps to identify triggers to agitation.

Preventing Agitation

1. Create a calm environment; remove stressors, triggers or danger. Move person to a safer or quieter place, offer rest and privacy, limit caffeine use; provide opportunity for exercise, develop soothing rituals, use gentle reminders
2. Avoid environmental triggers such as noise, glare, too much activity of background distraction
3. Check for pain, hunger, thirst, constipation, full bladder, fatigue, infections, and skin irritation. Check if temperature is comfortable, be sensitive to unspoken fears, misperceived threats, and frustration
4. Simplify tasks and routines
5. Allow for rest between stimulating activities
6. Use adequate lighting to reduce confusion at night.

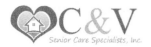

Identifying the Triggers

By identifying the trigger that has led to agitated behavior, the best behavioral intervention can be chosen. Often the trigger is some change in the person's environment such as:

1. Caregiver not recognizing their loved one is in pain
2. Change in caregiver
3. Change in living arrangements
4. Travel
5. Hospitalization
6. Presence of houseguests
7. Bathing
8. Being asked to change clothing

Responding to Agitation

1. Do: redirect individual's attention, back off; use calm positive statements, reassure, slow down, use visual and verbal cues, add light, offer guided choices between two options, focus on pleasant events, offer simple exercise options or limit stimulation

2. Do Not: raise your voice, take offense, corner the individual, crowd, restrain, rush, criticize, ignore, confront, argue, reason, shame, demand, condescend, force, explain, teach, show alarm, or move suddenly out of the person's view.

3. Things to Say: May I help you? Do you have time to help me? You are safe here. Everything is under control. I apologize. I am sorry that you are upset. I know it is hard. I will stay with you until you think better.

Making it safe

1. Equip doors and gates with safety locks
2. Make sure guns and other weapons are out of environment

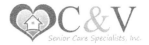

PARANOID and SUSPICIOUS BEHAVIOR

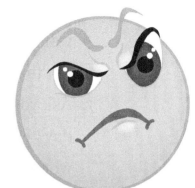

Because of memory loss and confusion, the individual with Alzheimer's disease may see things or interpret things incorrectly. The individual may become suspicious of those around him and accuse them of theft, infidelity, or improper behavior. The person may become paranoid or suspicious when he forgets where he put something and thinks others are taking her/his things, forgets his caregiver and sees the person as a stranger; does not know where he or she is or understand what instructions he or she is to follow. The paranoia is often a delusion. A delusion can be thought of as a false belief that, even in the light of contradictory evidence, remains fixed. The person with Alzheimer's genuinely believes the delusion is real. The caregiver, who spends many hours with him/her, is frequently accused of harming the person in some way. A person may think he or she is being poisoned, spied on, or items and money are being stolen.

What should you do?

1. Don't take offense – listen to what is troubling the individual and try to understand his/her reality. Then be reassuring and let the individual know that you care.
2. Don't try to argue or convince.
3. Offer a simple answer.
4. Switch the individual's attention to another activity or ask his/her help with a chore.

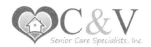

5. Duplicate items if lost. If individual is looking for a specific item, have several available. For example, the individual believes someone stole his wallet, purchase two of the same kind so you can produce the wallet and calm his/her fears.

6. Let the person know he or she is safe.

7. Ask yourself does suspicious behavior occur at certain times of the day? Does tiredness, poor lighting, isolation, and loneliness make it worse?

HOW TO HANDLE ACCUSATIONS OF STEALING:

EXAMPLE: A family member or patient you are caring for accuses you of stealing her purse. Take the following steps;

1-Count to 10. Calm yourself.

2-Say "Oh, Mrs. Jones you must feel terrible that you lost your purse" (VALIDATE HER FEELINGS)

3-"Mrs. Jones, let me help you find your purse". (OFFER TO HELP FIND THE PURSE)

4-"Mrs. Jones have you seen all the new fall fashions in the newspaper". (BEGIN TO USE DISTRACTION)

5. **KEEP TALKING FOR 5 MINUTES OR MORE**. (USE DISTRACTION, TAKING ADVANTAGE OF 5 MINUTES OF SHORT TERM MEMORY AND EVENTUALLY OFFERING A NEW ACTIVITY.)

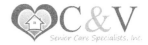

HOW TO HANDLE ACCUSATIONS OF CHEATING/INFIDELITY

When an individual with Alzheimer's accuses a spouse of cheating, it probably stems from fear that he/she will be abandoned by the spouse or other family members. This fear and resulting accusations can also arise because the person with Alzheimer's is beginning to have difficulty recognizing people and may interpret the actions of an acquaintance, who is no longer recognized, as the actions of someone who is "hitting on her/his spouse".

According to Geri R Hall, PhD, ARNP, GCNS, FAAN Clinical Nurse Specialist Banner Alzheimer's Institute in a CARING.COM blog she suggested the following technique when a spouse is dealing with accusations of cheating;

A. Acknowledge the individual's distress "You think I was cheating, oh Harold, I am so sorry your think that way. I will do anything you suggest to correct it!"

B. Apologize again: "I am so very sorry you think that. I love you and have no intention of leaving you. I will try to never upset you again."

C. Agree: "If I thought that you were cheating I would be as upset as you are."

D. Play dumb and promise to fix it....even cry a little. "Oh Harold, I don't know how this happened. I will make sure it never happens again. I'm here with you and have no plans to go anywhere."

E. Ask: Why don't we get some ice cream? What flavor would you like? (Ice cream is the great substitute for mood-controlling medications)

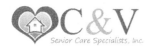

INAPPROPRIATE SEXUAL BEHAVIORS

Sexual behaviors are the most difficult to understand and to accept. These behaviors embarrass those that witness the behaviors and lead to further isolation of the individual. The following are examples of hypersexual behavior:

1. Compulsive masturbation in both public and private locations
2. A pattern of lewd, suggestive language
3. Fondling of breasts or other private body parts of caregivers as well as strangers
4. Flirtation
5. Disrobing of self or others, and
6. Overt sexual acts
7. "Coming on" to adult children- confusing them for a "younger version" of spouse

Hypersexual behavior is typically directed at a number of people, not one particular relationship. Hyper-sexuality is not a form of sexual intimacy that may be retained in Alzheimer's disease. The reasons for hyper-sexuality are very complex. Generally it is believed that the behavior is due to chemical and physical changes in the brain. There are also suggested psychological causes such as loss of self-esteem and self-image and lack of physical closeness.

Sometimes what we think is inappropriate sexual behavior may mean something else. For instance, if someone is removing his clothing, it may be that the shirt is uncomfortable, or the tag in the back is irritating. If a male individual exposes his penis or masturbates it may mean that he needs to go

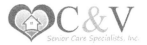

to the bathroom. If you can't figure out why the individual is removing clothing or exposing self, cover the person with a butcher's apron. If the individual can't get to the clothing, the problem stops. What appears to be a sexual behavior may also relate to a symptom of Alzheimer's called visual agnosia – the inability to comprehend what they see. So when the individual urinates in the trash can or sink it may well be because they misinterpreted the trash can and the sink as the toilet.

What Can We Do? Traditional interventions should be attempted before medication. One basic need of persons exhibiting hyper-sexuality is the need for connections with others. These needs may be able to be met in ways such as conversation, taking a walk, sitting having a snack or drink with someone. This is an area that families need to be aware of so that they are prepared when and if these behaviors occur. As a last resort, a consultation with the physician regarding the benefits of medication to deal with hyper-sexuality may be necessary. One of the most promising medications for this problem is the SSRIs – Selective Serotonin Reuptake Inhibitors- generally used for depression. These medications tend to decrease libido with few side effects.

However as the disease progresses, many individuals with Alzheimer's disease become active masturbators. We may think uncomfortable but we just have to accept it. It is one of the few pleasures they have left. So if the individual begins to masturbate simply remove the individual to a private area.

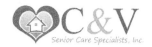

AFFIRMING POSITIVE BEHAVIORS

Even though the person with dementia has significant memory loss and decline in intellectual function, this does not mean that the need for affection and comfort has disappeared. In fact, when the world becomes a strange and confusing place, the person's needs for support and affection become even more important.

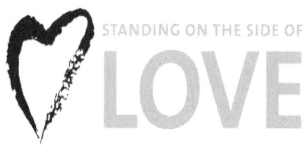

It is easy to slip into a way of thinking that is negative and focuses on "ain't it awful". Once in a while you can allow yourself to have an "ain't it awful" cry. But it is not a good idea to remain in this place. It is not good for you or the person for whom you provide care. So once you allow yourself this time, then you need to make a conscious effort to "catch the person being good". Every time something goes well – the person eats his food, drinks all of his juice, allows you to assist in bathing, he/she wipes the table clean, and he/she folds the laundry, then offer praise. Tell the person how grateful you are, and if this is your loved one, tell him how much you love him and give him a hug. Remember that Alzheimer's disease steals

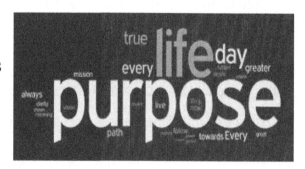

memories; it does not steal the emotions that make memories come alive. The emotions are still there and they still need to be nurtured.

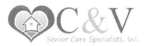

NURTURING THE SPIRIT: THE IMPORTANCE OF SPIRITUAL/RELIGIOUS INTERVENTIONS

It is important to provide spiritual experiences for the individual. For many individuals long after the ability to speak is gone, they still respond to religious music, religious services and other religious or spiritual practices.

"Profound memory loss is associated with 'loss of self'. However, it never means loss of soul! As providers we must be aware of how memory loss can lead to chaos in the soul. Our memories allow us to hold onto God's loving presence in our lives. We can trust in God to be present to us in the here and now only because we remember the experience of God's presence and help in our past.

The person with AD experiences a break in the very memories that provide continuity and connection to God that sustains most of us until our last breath. For a person with AD every day is new and everyone is a stranger —with no connection to the past, how can the person with AD experience trust that God will not abandon him? When one cannot remember who one is it is difficult to remember whose one is (God's) and to find comfort.

Buckwalter, G. (2003). Addressing the Spiritual and Religious Needs of Persons with Profound Memory Loss. *Home Healthcare Nurse.* 21(1), 20-21.

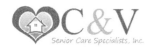

Each of us that touch this individual's life – caregivers as well as the community of faith- have a responsibility to assist the person with AD to find his/her way home to God through the chaos and confusion of dementia. In order to carry out this responsibility and privilege it is essential that we discover the individual's

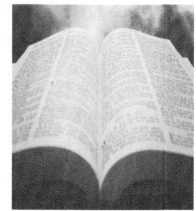

"meaning making" history. This history may lead us to use religious music, religious symbols, as well as rituals to reach the individual but the history may also lead us to use art, photography, and nature to make connections.

The use of visual aids such as a Bible, rosary, candles, mezuzahs, menorahs, sculptures of praying hands, the use of sounds, such as

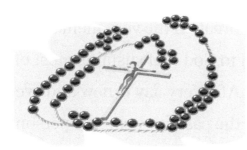

recordings of hymns, organs, the shofar horn, words of Scripture, liturgy, as well as smells such as incense, fresh bread, and wine are all life giving and provide bridges that assist the person with AD to reconnect the person with AD to body memories that create a positive spiritual and emotional affect.

It is important to strengthen the pastoral connection that the individual has to his church/synagogue/mosque. A visit from a priest, minister, rabbi, or Imam can provide powerful spiritual comfort.

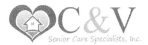

Reception of the sacraments remains an important spiritual event for Christian individuals with AD.

Role of Parish or Faith Community Nurse: There are a growing number of nurses who are associated with faith communities. These nurses are invaluable resources in making sure that the spiritual needs of a loved one with Alzheimer's are met. Check this out with your place of worship to see if there is a nurse on board and if there is make contact with this nurse and inform her/him that you have a loved one who has spiritual needs. Or just as important that you would love to attend worship services if you either had someone who could stay with your loved one and/or provide you with transportation.

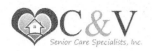

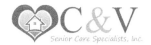

SECTION 7

SPECIAL CONSIDERATIONS

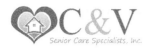

VALUE OF MUSIC

Have you ever heard a song playing on the radio and found yourself transported to a time and place from the past? Have you ever had a song stir your deepest emotions – and bring back memories as if those experiences were happening in the present? Have you ever been comforted, stimulated, saddened, elated or experienced some other powerful emotion just because of a song? Most of us have had such experiences and the power of the "remembering" elicited by music can catch us "off guard" when the song evokes emotionally charged memories. Music has the same power with individuals diagnosed with Alzheimer's and knowing this provides one more tool to help family as well as paid caregivers to manage challenging behaviors, to reach someone who appears to be lost in the disease, to calm an agitated individual, to encourage cooperation in activities such as bathing that might otherwise be met with resistance. Some research even indicates that music can help restore lost memories and bring those afflicted with the disease back into the present – if only for a short period of time.

These facts about the power of music seem to fly in the face of the progressive loss of memories associated with Alzheimer's disease– starting with the most recent and steadily erasing long ago memories going back in time. However it is important to know that memories of music are "wired" differently in the brain than other memories – it is almost as if the brain is made to contain music. Whereas short term memories are stored in the Hippocampus, music is stored everywhere in the brain and music with all of its emotional meanings continues to be accessible to people with Alzheimer's even when they have lost the ability to speak – many can still sing!

What a powerful idea this is! If caregivers fully appreciated the significance of music they would use it all the time and to facilitate many activities of daily living. Caregivers have shared that they engage the person with Alzheimer's in singing while the individual is bathed and dressed. Nurses sometimes use music while they are performing a painful procedure such as dressing a wound or drawing blood – music can distract, can soothe and can engage the person with Alzheimer's disease.

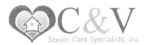

A research study conducted by Brandon Ally an assistant professor at Boston University, where 32 Alzheimer's individuals participated in a research study that examined the power of music and found that these subjects were able to learn more lyrics when the words were set to music than when they were spoken. Ally believes that the results of this study suggest that those with Alzheimer's could be helped to remember things that are both necessary to their independence and well-being. For instance, creating a short ditty about taking medications or the importance of brushing one's teeth might be a strategy to help those with AD maintain abilities to perform these necessary skills. This was the first study to demonstrate that using music can help people with Alzheimer's to learn new information through the use of music (Seligson, S, June 15, 2010 *http://www.bu.edu/today/2010/music-boosts-memory-in-alzheimer%E2%80%99s/*)

In the famous U-Tube *Man In Nursing Home Reacts To Hearing Music From His Era* we see Henry, a man who was almost totally unresponsive begin to respond with sound, movement and facial animation when he uses an I-Pod programmed with "Henry's music" . After the I-pod is removed Henry is not only quite spirited but totally involved in the ensuing conversation. He is able to discuss his favorite musician, Cab Calloway, and when asked "what is your favorite Cab Calloway song?" Henry begins to sing "I'll be home for Christmas". Not only is his speech perfectly clear, his face is expressive, he uses his hands in explaining the emotional power of music. The interviewer inquires of Henry "what does Cab Calloway's music mean to you? Henry talks about what music does for him – that the Good Lord changed him through music and made him a "holy man". The transformation of Henry is nothing short of miraculous and raises questions about why music is not used in every home where someone with Alzheimer's is cared for, in every Assisted Living Facility and in every Skilled Nursing Home (*http://www.youtube.com/watch?v=fyZQfop73QM*).

Music should be a routine part of care – not only does it bring joy to the person with this terrible disease, it allows for continuing connections between the caregiver and the person with AD. It diminishes the lonely isolation that is part of the disease when the afflicted person appears to be locked in a world that is isolated and isolating to others.

One more story about the power of music. A gentleman named Ben shared this story about his wife who had been diagnosed with Alzheimer's and was well into the middle stage when he placed her in a facility for care. Ben visited often

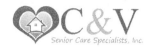

and one of the techniques he used to stay connected to his wife and to make the visits pleasant and meaningful for both of them was to draw on his wife's past history with music. She had sung for many years with the Sweet Adeline's and she retained her lovely singing voice despite the ravages of Alzheimer's disease. Ben loaded music that his wife had sung throughout her years with the Sweet Adeline's, he attached two sets of earphones – one set for his wife and one set for himself and they would sing together. Music was a powerful connection between them that remained until his wife passed away.

Music is so important – the power of music to maintain connections, relationships and joy in life cannot be over emphasized

Seligson, S, June 15, 2010 *http://www.bu.edu/today/2010/music-boosts-memory-in-alzheimer%E2%80%99s/* Accessed July 8, 2012

Man In Nursing Home Reacts To Hearing Music From His Era (April 2012). (*http://www.youtube.com/watch?v=fyZQfop73QM*) *www.youtube.com* Accessed July 8, 2012

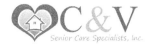

HOLIDAY CELEBRATIONS

When caring for a loved one with Alzheimer's disease (AD) the holidays may also be stressful, sad and overwhelming. Caregivers of those with this disease may think that holiday preparation is more than he or she is capable of handling. Individuals with the disease may find much that accompanies traditional celebrations to be overwhelming, stressful and confusing. As caregivers we need to take a look at traditions to determine what they are still able to maintain and what they can easily let go. We can also help caregivers to find ways to make the holidays as pleasant and stress free as possible for the person with AD. Preparation is the key to success in this area.

The problems arise when the person with AD is in the middle stage of the disease, functioning somewhere between the level of a 4 year old deteriorating to that of a two year old. When we are raising small children between these ages we are keenly aware that much that goes into holiday celebrations is upsetting to small children. Disruptions to their normal routines of nap and meal times may result in difficult behaviors. Sometimes they are overwhelmed by the numbers of people surrounding them; the increased noise and confusion is difficult for them to bear. So too the person with Alzheimer's may find the holidays overwhelming, resulting in difficult behaviors.

It is important for families who are caring for a loved one with AD to modify expectations regarding the holidays. This can best be accomplished by calling for a face-to- face meeting or conference call with family and friends to discuss how Alzheimer's has impacted both the person with the disease as well as the primary caregiver and immediate family. It is unrealistic for the primary caregiver to maintain every holiday tradition while at the same time he/she is providing care. The caregiver needs to give her/himself permission to simplify,

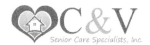

simplify, simplify! For example, if the tradition has been to host a sit-down dinner for 20 – perhaps the new tradition involves inviting immediate family for a simple meal or for everyone participating in the meal to bring a favorite dish.

Furthermore it makes sense to inform those who are not intimately aware of the situation to write or call them so they are prepared for the changes that have occurred in the person with AD. The Alzheimer's Association suggests that the caregiver share ahead of time that the loved one with AD may display challenging behaviors, may not remember the names of visitors and may confuse them with others, and that the person with AD may have changed in appearance. Sharing a picture or a description of the changes is helpful so that visitors do not appear shocked or "put- off" by the changes. Visitors should be coached to provide their names and relationships to the person with AD, with statements such as "Hi, I am your cousin Rob – we used to have such fun together when we were children." Visitors should be cautioned against asking "Do you remember who I am?" Questions like this only make the person with AD think more confused and anxious about his/her memory problems. Another intervention would be to provide adhesive backed name tags so that everyone who enters the home writes on the name tags their name and relationship to the person with AD. Reading ability remains until late in the middle stage and is a strategy that allows the person with AD to be able to read "cheat sheets" that ease her/his anxiety when faced with people that he/she thinks should be recognizable yet recalling names is impossible.

The individual with AD needs to participate in holiday preparations as much as his/her abilities allow. For instance, the person might be able to help in the kitchen doing repetitive activities like mixing cookie dough, washing or peeling

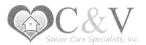

fresh vegetables or setting the table; they might be able to participate in wrapping presents (the caregiver needs to be tolerant of "less than perfect" results). It is important that the caregiver is aware of maintaining the loved one's routine as much as possible. Without this awareness, holiday preparation can become confusing and disruptive to the person with AD. Building on past traditions that draw on "old memories" are wonderful things to do – activities such as singing old holiday songs might be both comforting as well as fun for both the caregiver as well as for the person receiving care. Encouraging the person with AD to watch old movies that are holiday classics such as *It's a Good Life* or *Miracle on 34th Street* are a way to fill time in a pleasant manner.

Gift giving can be another challenge when caring for someone with AD. Those who want to give gifts could benefit from some simple directions such as buying useful items such as an ID bracelet (available through MedicAlert® and the Alzheimer's Association Safe Return® program), fleece lined sweat pants and tops that are easy to put on and because they are lined with fleece remain soft and non-irritating to the individual's skin; memory books, photo albums, the Video Respite Series available on-line from the Best Alzheimer's Products' – these are all gifts that will benefit both the person with Alzheimer's as well as her/his caregiver. The individual with AD may still enjoy giving gifts. For example if the individual used to bake, assisting her/him to make cookies and helping the individual to pack them into tins or boxes may be an activity that allows the person to think "part-of" the festivities.

Flexibility is also essential when planning holiday activities – keeping in mind the needs of the person with AD. For instance if the person with AD experiences sun-downing or evening confusion, it makes sense to plan all

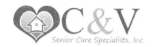

celebrations earlier in the day when the person with AD is at her/his best. The primary caregiver needs to be cognizant of her/his own needs and builds in "away" time with others. Engaging the services of others to provide "in—home" care allows the caregiver the freedom to enjoy some time without the constant demands of caregiving.

References: Alzheimer's Association (2007). Holidays.

Terrazas, B. (2010). How to Cope with Alzheimer's during the Holidays. *Dallas News;* http://dallasnews.com/health/headlines/20101108-How-to-cope-with-Alzheimer-s8324.ece. *Accessed 10/17/2011.*

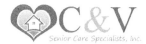

VACATIONS AND CAR TRAVELING

A caregiver to someone with Alzheimer's disease (AD) who is planning a vacation needs to be aware that a vacation may not be the restful and relaxing get away that the caregiver has in mind when planning such a trip. Vacations do not "relax" the person with Alzheimer's and on the contrary may precipitate a catastrophic reaction in that individual. The person with memory deficits may function sufficiently well in a familiar situation where he/she is not challenged to respond to unfamiliar places, persons, situations and a different schedule for the day. However, a vacation disrupts all of that "sameness" and familiarity, plunging the person into situations that are not only unfamiliar but potentially very frightening. Home health care providers may be called on for advice regarding strategies to make a vacation not only pleasant but safe both for the person with AD but also for the caregiver.

Certainly an individual's reaction to a vacation is greatly impacted by the degree of decline that has occurred due to Alzheimer's. A 'great fooler' still in the early stage of the disease will probably be able to handle the changes that accompany a vacation with relative ease. However for someone in the middle stage, functioning at the cognitive level of a toddler, 4 years old deteriorating to 2 years old, a vacation could be stressful for everyone involved. In fact the answer for a caregiver who desires to take a vacation, might be to consider placing the person with AD in respite care –which is available either through some home health care agencies where a professional caregiver stays in the home while the caregiver is away, through assisted living facilities or by bringing into the home, a familiar individual, a friend or family member, to provide care so that the person with AD remains in her/his home following familiar routines.

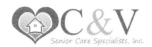

However if the caregiver decides that including the loved one with Alzheimer's is worth the effort involved in the planning, there are certainly steps to take in preparation for a trip that will lessen the stress and make the vacation safer. Taking a short "test" trip might be a good idea to see how the person with AD reacts to traveling. Planning the vacation destination for a location that is familiar to the person with AD and avoiding places that are over-crowded are also good strategies to consider. If the vacation includes visiting relatives and/or friends who are not aware of the changes that have occurred in the person with AD, it makes sense to forewarn those individuals about what to expect. For instance, informing them that Sam still likes to use his hands to build things but "these days he focuses on manipulating and building with "Legos" gives them a "heads up" regarding Sam's condition. If the person with AD is a wanderer, it is essential that he/she is enrolled in the Alzheimer's Association's Safe Return Program and that he/she wears an identification bracelet before embarking to a different locale. If the vacation involves flying and/or staying in a hotel it is also important for the caregiver to inform the airline and hotel staff that she/he is traveling with a memory impaired individual.

The caregiver needs to take into account the needs of the person with AD. For instance, what are the bathroom needs of the individual – is the person incontinent and if so how will this be handled on a trip? Packing ample incontinent products, wipes and changes of clothing that are easily accessible if needed is an important consideration. Beverly Bigtree Murphy (*http://bigtreemurphy.com, Accessed July 11, 2012*) created a website that includes practical and easy to use strategies for dealing with incontinence during automobile travel. Bigtree-Murphy suggests if traveling by car to look for service stations along main highways. These facilities usually have a single

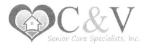

occupancy bathroom that not only provide privacy but will also have a sink that allows for clean-up from a bowel movement. This allows greater privacy for both the caregiver and the recipient of care. Major rest stops are usually equipped with multi-stall units with a sink outside of where the toilets are located.

Packing needs to focus not only on changes of clothing but also on bringing enough prescribed as well as "over the counter" medications to deal with the unexpected physical issues that might arise such as diarrhea or constipation, headache, and an upset stomach. Additionally, the planning for a trip needs to take into account activities that the person with AD can participate in while traveling. For instance, loading an IPod with music that the individual loves, bringing along a deck of cards so that the person can either engage in a card game or for some individuals just holding and manipulating cards might be soothing.

If possible there should be at least an additional person in the car who can focus on keeping the individual with AD calm, occupied and safely seat-belted. The itinerary for the trip needs to include regular rest stops. If the caregiver is traveling alone with the person with AD and the individual with Alzheimer's becomes agitated, it is important for the caregiver to stop the car and to attend to the person's needs-driving while trying to calm an agitated individual is a disaster in the offing.

Clearly vacations are possible – but taking one involves considerable planning on the part of the caregiver.

- Reference: Bigtree-Murphy, B. (2000). *Incontinence: Everything You Need to Know and Hoped You'd Never Have to Ask! Accessed July 11, 2012, http://bigtreemurphy.com*

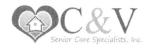

HOW TO RESPOND TO CHIDREN'S QUESTIONS

Invariably young children, faced with a grandparent who is changing because of Alzheimer's, ask "what's wrong with grandma or grandpa? Children need explanations. They are attuned to the emotional climate that they live in and sensitive to signs that their parents are worried or upset. Without an explanation of what is going on, children will assume that they are responsible for the tension in the home and that they have done something to make mommy and daddy upset. The first step is to explain to children that Alzheimer's is a disease that changes the way grandma or grandpa acts and makes her/him forget things. The details that are provided to the child depend on the child's age. For instance, it makes sense to tell a child that Alzheimer's is an illness that changes Grandma's brain in the inside. Grandma may look the same on the outside but her brain is slowly changing from the inside. These changes lead to forgetting lots of important things including people, even very important and loved people like grandchildren.

Children will need reminders when the grandparent displays challenging behaviors that grandma or grandpa is really ill. If children are witnesses to catastrophic reactions where grandma is crying and/or screaming, it is a common response that these children will assume that they have done something wrong that made grandma behave in this way. It is not unusual for children to carry an enormous burden of undeserved guilt and feel responsible for behaviors for which they bear no responsibility. They need reassurance, repeated explanations that grandma is sick, that she loves them, and that they remain an important part of her life.

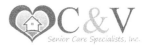

Sometimes children are the targets of accusations of stealing or other wrongdoing, because grandma lacks the memory of where she placed her purse or her keys. Out of her own frustration she blames any and all those around her for stealing. These accusations are difficult for adult family members to accept and even more difficult for children to handle. Very young children require comfort and consolation and assurance that they are not to blame. School age children and older can be taught how to respond to grandma in a helpful manner. The following technique requires practice with the parent but results in defusing accusations and communicating love to grandma. The technique involves using the technique of validation that grandma is upset because she lost her purse, slowly changing the subject (using the knowledge that grandma only has about five minutes of short term memory) and relying on the power of distraction to move away from the false accusation.

Rather than verbally denying wrong doing the child might say, *"Oh Grandma I am so sorry that your purse is missing…please don't worry – I will help you find it. When I lost my favorite doll I was so upset and you helped me find it. I will help you find your purse. Let's look for it together. I am sure it is somewhere – we just have to look. Where have you looked for it? Did you search in the closet? Under the bed? I remember that we found my doll underneath the dining room table. Have you looked there?"* The child is then taught to change the subject, *"Grandma did I tell you about my school trip? We went to a farm and picked apples. We watched the people at the farm make apple butter. It was so much fun and it made me think of all the good things that you used to cook."* This strategy of validating, offering to help and changing the subject is a powerfully effective one that school age children can master.

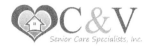

Children may worry that their parents are going to "catch" Alzheimer's like they catch colds from others. They need reassurance that Alzheimer's is an illness that is not spread from one person to another and that most people don't get this disease. It is important for children to be told that grandma will have good days and bad days and that the routines in the home might change. Most importantly children need to be told that they are loved – no matter what the circumstances of grandma's illness.

It is important to encourage conversation about grandma. The parents need to open the conversation by asking children about their own observations about grandma; have they noticed anything that she really likes or that seems to make her smile? Have they noticed any changes in grandma and how do they think about the changes they are seeing? Helping children to talk openly about their own feelings, worries and fears allows the parent to reassure and to let the children know that the feelings are normal – in fact the parent experiences similar feelings.

Sometimes children express their emotions in indirect ways. A child may complain of "not feeling good" but not be able to pinpoint what is wrong. School performance might show a decline. Children may be hesitant to invite friends to their home because they are afraid of what grandma might say or do. These behaviors need to be gently confronted while offering the child comfort and support.

It is important to help children stay involved with grandma. They can be encouraged to set the table together, by looking at picture albums, listening to music, dancing or any simple activity that can be shared. It is important for parents to help children find ways to interact with their grandparent. Lastly to

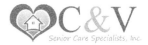

assist children in their understanding of Alzheimer's it is helpful for parents to read to their children age-appropriate books on the disease. There are a number of excellent books on the market. For instance, *What's Happening to Grandpa" (2004)* written by Maria Shriver is a sad but wonderful book based on her experiences with her own father who died from Alzheimer's disease; *Always my Grandpa: A story for Children about Alzheimer's Disease,* written by Linda Scacco and Nicole Woy in 2005 and *Still My Grandma,* written by Veronique Van Den Abeele and Claude Dubois in 2007 are also wonderful books and assist parents in explaining this terrible disease that slowly takes Grandma or Grandpa away.

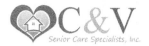

MANAGING YOUR LOVED ONE FROM A DISTANCE

Caring or assisting to care for a loved one with Alzheimer's or a related dementia isn't easy. Living a distance from your loved one can complicate caregiving. One can think overwhelmed with managing health care, safety, nutrition, finances and the loved one's home.

There are several simple strategies to manage a loved one from a distance that can be helpful. What is important to know up front is where your loved one is in his/her progression through the disease. Depending on what stage the person is in will dictate what level of care you need to provide. Someone in the early stage can function with reminders and be left alone for periods of time. Early in the middle stage when the person is functioning cognitively at a toddler level, it is not safe to leave the person with Alzheimer's alone. The person will need supervision round the clock. In the late stage, care will be more intensive and hands on as there may be little your loved one can do independently.

IDENTIFY HELP NEEDED TO

MAINTAIN YOUR LOVED ONE AT HOME

1. Determine what services you will need assistance in providing care to your loved one.

    - Health Care (Physicians, Home Care, Assistive Devices)
    - Meals/Food
    - Legal
    - Financial
    - Medicine
    - Bills
    - Safety & House Maintenance

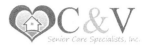

2. Who will be with your loved one? Who will make sure she/he is safe?
   Remember where your loved one is in her/his progression in the disease –
   this will help you determine how much care you need for your loved one.

   A) Family members, friends?

   B) Home Care-Does your loved need someone to assist them with personal
      care or medical care? Medication management? Acute or chronic disease
      management?

   C) Aging services - *www.eldercare.gov*

   D) Community Agencies-Meals on Wheels, Aging Organizations, County
      Senior Services, Respite services?

   E) Durable Medical Equipment for needed assistive devices such as
      walkers, canes, ramps, lifts

   F) Lifeline or Emergency Alert Services?

   G) Support in managing financial and legal issues?

3. Who will oversee her/his day to day care?

   A) Family, friends?

   B) Geriatric Care Manager-Is a social worker or a nurse who can be hired
      to oversee some or all of your loved one's care? A Care manager in your
      area can be found by going to *www.caremanager.org*

   C) Primary Care Physician-Supportive of efforts to maintain your loved
      one at home?

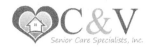

ESTABLISH A CONTACT LIST OF SUPPORTS FOR

YOUR LOVED ONE

(HAVE A PHONE DIRECTORY, SO ALL CAREGIVERS KNOW CONTACTS)

1. Relatives, friends' numbers

    a. House Maintenance-Who can provide services such as mowing the lawn, and home maintenance and repairs?

2. Physicians involved in your loved one's care

3. Assistive devices-local DME providers, *http://alzstore .com*

4. Home Care – list of providers who can assist with personal care, bathing and providers who can provide medical   skilled services. *www.nahc.org*

5. Geriatric Care Manager-Call the Association of Professional Geriatric Care Managers at 1-520-881-8008 or *www.caremanagers .org*

6. Legal Professional - Lawyer who maintains wills, handles power of attorney and can assist with legal, financial and healthcare decisions. To find an elder law attorney, go to *www.neala org*.

7. Banking – Know who can handle banking responsibilities. Know the rules of your loved ones bank.

8. Pharmacies - (do any deliver?)

9. Lifeline (Emergency Alert Systems)

10. Community organizations - church, faith community resources, volunteer groups, Aging services, senior services

11. Transportation

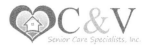

MAKE THE MOST OF YOUR VISITS WITH

YOUR LOVED ONE

1   Check in with family and professional caregivers to see how your loved one is doing. Praise these caregivers for their patience and time spent. Give them needed respite as time allows.

2   Make appointments prior to the visit to take your loved one to the doctor, lawyer, shopping. Make appointments with caregivers, legal or financial managers to modify any needed matters.

3   Schedule some leisure time together –share a meal, reminisce with a photo album, take a car ride, plan a picnic at home. Make sure to try to maintain your loved one's routines.

4   Prepare meals, buy supplies for the house, organize and clean house. Fill prescriptions.

KEEP IN CONTACT WITH YOUR LOVED ONE

1   Call to say "hello." Introduce yourself. Don't make your loved one guess who is calling. Don't quiz them. You are not calling to test their memory but to check-in with them to let them know you are thinking about them.

2   Write letters and send pictures. Label the pictures with the names of who is in the photo and where the photo was taken from vacation, home, etc.

3   Create albums for your loved one of you and your family.

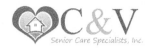

ADDITIONAL RESOURCES

In addition to the resources you find in this booklet there are so many others that are available through the Alzheimer's Association, through the government, and through ADEAR (Alzheimer's Disease Education and Resource). If you have access to a computer at home then resource information is available at your fingertips and most of it is free! If you don't have that access, take a trip to your local library to access this invaluable educational support.

ALZHEIMER'S WEBSITES

1   The Alzheimer's Association (*www.Alz.org*) is a national group that provides:

- Free educational materials printable in your own home;

- Caregiver support groups where you can meet others whose experiences mirror your own—there is great value in knowing you are not alone.

- Respite—many of the local chapters of the Alzheimer's Association provide limited and free respite care so you can get away for a few hours or even longer.

- Safe Return Program (see in this resource guide)

- Telephone support if you are feeling "at the end of your rope" as a caregiver

- Annual Alzheimer's Walk

- Lending library of teaching videos – available for individual as well as group use.

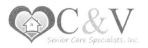

2   Alzheimer's Disease Education and Referral Center (ADEAR). Available at: *http://www.nia.nih.gov/alzheimers* Get some of their great resources updated "Hospitalization Happens: A Guide to Hospital Visits for Individuals with Memory Loss." And "Caring for a Person with Alzheimer's disease; Your Easy-to-Use Guide"**800-438-4380**

3   Alzheimer's Foundation of America. Available at: *http://www.alzfdn.org*

4   Association for Frontotemporal Dementias Available at:

http://www.theaftf.org

5   Family Caregiver Alliance. Available at: *http://www.caregiver .com*

6   National Family Caregivers Association.   Available at

http://www.thefamilycaregiver .org

7   A Caregiver's Guide to Alzheimer's Disease. Available at:

http://www.medical-assistant.net/Alzheimer's-resources

8   Cognitive Dynamics. Available at: http://www.cognitivedynamics.org

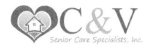

GREAT DOWNLOADS

1. Frank Broyle's Playbook for Alzheimer's Caregivers is an excellent, practical and easy read for caregivers. It is **FREE** and can be ordered or down loaded for print at: *www.alzheimersplaybook .com* .

The book is a football themed, practical guide that addresses, "Pre-Game Planning," "Coaches and Special Teams," "Playing Offense," and "The Training Table" for each stage of the disease.

In addition to these resources there is a wealth of written information— biographical as well as autobiographical accounts from caregivers as well as from those who are journeying through the disease—who want to share with others not only their experiences but the joys that are possible.

PHYSICIAN AND CAREGIVER RESOURCES FOR DRIVERS WITH DEMENTIA

- Eldercare (*http://www.eldercare.gov*)

- AAA Foundation for Traffic Safety (*http://www.aaafoundation.org*)

- Senior Driving (*http://www.seniordrivers .org*)

- Community Transportation Association (*http://www.ctaa .org/ntrc/seniorpublications .asp*)

- American Public Transportation Association (*http://www.publictransportation .org/systems/*)

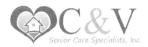

- Easter Seals (*http://www.easter-seals.org/ntltranscare*)

- NationalAssociation of Area Agencies on Aging (*http://www.n4a.org*)

- NationalHighway Traffic Safety Administration (*http://www.nhtsa.dot.gov/people/injury/olddrive/*)

- American Occupational Therapy Association (*http://www.aota.org/olderdriver*)

- Association for Driver Rehabilitation Specialists (*http://www.aded.net*)

- American Medical Association (*http://www.ama-assn.org/go/olderdrivers*)

- Administration on Aging (*http://www.aoa.gov*)

Adapted from Carr D, Rebok GW. *The Older Adult Driver.* In: Gallo JJ, Bogner, HR, Fulmer T., Pareza GJ, eds. *Handbook of Geriatric Assessment.*4th ed. Boston: Jones and Bartlett, 2005:53 .

BOOKS

- *The 36–Hour Day: A Family Guide to Caring for Persons With Alzheimer Disease Related Dementing Illnesses, and Memory Loss in Later Life.* Nancy L. Mace and Peter V. Rabins, Mass Market Paperback, 2001

- *Learning to Speak Alzheimer's: A Groundbreaking Approach for Everyone Dealing with the Disease.* Joanne Koenig Coste and Robert Butler, Mariner Books, 2003

- *Alzheimer's Disease: What If There Was a Cure?* Mary T. Newport, Basic Health Publications, 2011.

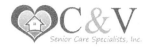

- *Caregiver Survival Series*. Sherman, James R .Pathway Books, 1997

- *Preventing Caregiver Burnout* (1997).

- *Creating Moments of Joy: A Journal for Caregivers*, Fourth Edition Jolene Brackey, Purdue University Press, 2007.

- *Creative Caregiving* (1997).

- *Coping With Caregiving Worries* (1997).

- *The Caregiver's Handbook: A Complete Guide to Home Health Care*. Visiting Nurse Associations of America, DK Publishing, 1998.

- *The Caregiver's Manual*. Williams, G .and Kay, P. Citadel Press, 1995.

- *Caregiving: The Spiritual Journey of Love, Loss, and Renewal*. McLeod, B. John Wiley and Sons, Inc.,1999.

- *Comfort of Home: An Illustrated Step–by–Step Guide for Caregivers*. Meyer, M. with Derr, P. Care Trust Publications, 1999.

- *Counting on Kindness: The Dilemmas of Dependency*. Lustbader, W. The Free Press, 1994.

- *Helping Yourself Help Others: A Book for Caregivers*. Carter, R. Random House, 1994.

- *Hiring Home Caregivers: The Family Guide to In–Home Eldercare*. Susik, D. Impact Publishers/American Source Books,1995

- *The Hospice Handbook*. Beresford, L .Little Brown and Co.,1993.

- *Kind Words for Caring People: Daily Affirmations for Caregivers*. Pitzele, S. Health Communications, 1992.

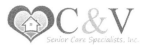

- *Share the Care.* Capossela,C., Warnock, S. Fireside Books/Simon & Schuster, 1995

- *Taking Charge: Overcoming the Challenges of Long–Term Illness.* Pollin, I. with Golant, S. Times Books, 1994.

- *Taking Time for Me: How Caregivers Can Effectively Deal With Stress.* Karr, K. Prometheus Books, 1992.

FINANCIAL PLANNING AND ALZHEIMER's

- *Financial Planning: a key but neglected part of Alzheimer's care.* University of California Health: *http://ucsf.edu/financialplanning.com*

- *Financial Planning and Alzheimer's/Dementia.* Jane Nowak: *http://moneygal2020.worldpress.com/category/healthcare*

- *Financial Planning for a Loved One Diagnosed with an Illness.* Financial Planning Association: *http://plannerssearch.org/pages/homeaspx*

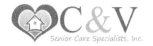

VIDEOS

1) Dementia with Dignity

A guide to caring for people with Alzheimer's disease. For colleges, nursing homes and home carers of dementia.

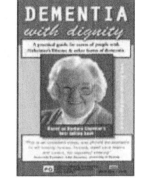

This popular "hands on "training video, based on Barbara Sherman's internationally - acclaimed book of the same name, is used world-wide. Filmed on location in residential and day care facilities in Australia, this program is relevant to all caregivers – in residential facilities, community care and family homes. An initiative of Media One and author Barbara Sherman, it was produced in conjunction with Eastway Communication, with executive consultants:

Training and Resource Centre for Residential Aged Care. The video can be obtained by going to: *www.terranova.org* purchase price is $169 .00. There are other excellent videos available on the Terranova website—but this is the most comprehensive one.

2) There is a Bridge by searching: *www.memorybridge .org* – a phenomenal video that emphasizes the truth that there is always a person we can reach, touch, communicate with and connect with

IT IS NEVER TRUE THAT THE "SELF" OF THE PERSON WITH AD IS GONE! The video costs $34 .95+S&H

Made in the USA
Monee, IL
18 May 2023

33994235R00070